THE BOOK ON HEALTHCARE IT

What you need to know about HIPAA, Hospital IT, and Healthcare Information Technology

JAMES SCOTT

THE BOOK ON HEALTHCARE IT

CONTENTS

PREFACE

This book truly simplifies the complicated and multifaceted topic of Healthcare IT with all its various niche terms and subjects such as HIPAA, Hospital IT, HITECH, Healthcare Information Technology, HIT etc. The overly technical jargon and robotic language has been virtually eliminated so that anyone with an interest in the topic of Health IT will find it easy to read and understand the terms being tossed around in the industry today. After reading only a few charters in the manual you will see why it stands out among IT resources in the Healthcare Books section.

This book cuts through the confusion and delivers a powerful explanation in a simplified manner, offering optimized comprehension of this complicated topic. Don't mistake simplification for limited delivery of quality content. This text covers the hot topics such as: options for encryption of personal health information, best ways to protect patient privacy, HIPAA requirements and compliance, prevention of fraud by healthcare insiders, wireless network security do's and don'ts and even a section on what we can learn from the Catholic Health System's network and data security.

This book is a crash course on the most common issues hospitals, medical record handlers and Healthcare IT professionals face on a daily basis. The author structures the topics in a manner that defines the issue and explains the easiest and most effective path from point A to point B so that the reader can better comprehend the actions necessary for a desirable outcome that both protects the hospital, patient data and healthcare professionals.

Minimizing risks, cybersecurity and patient privacy are at the core of discussions in the healthcare industry. This book offers the express learning bridge that has been missing in the industry until now.

THE MEDIOCRITY OF HEALTHCARE IT SECURITY

According to experts, healthcare organizations and their business associates are not doing a good enough job with information security.

After the ruling of the HIPPA Omnibus, experts are finding that healthcare organizations and their business associates have a long way to go in terms of tackling the fundamentals in information system programs. This is the assessment of several consultants in an informal survey of security and privacy experts. Most of them give only an average grade at best to the state of information security at healthcare units and the business associates providing service to these organizations.

WHAT ARE THE WEAK SPOTS?

According to experts, the most common weak spots are the fundamental but vital aspects that are needed for a strong program of information security: thorough risk assessments done in a timely manner, documented procedures and policies as well as relevant training of the workforce. Appropriate focus on these areas could vastly improve the grade of information security programs.

The Office for Civil Rights (OCR) enforces HIPAA. A former senior advisor says there is significant variability within OCR as well as other private sectors, based on the scope, size and commitment of the organization to secure health information. While some organizations are making an all-out effort in their programs to secure patient data, unfortunately that is not the case for all.

At some of the other organizations, although of the same type and size, leadership seems to only be interested in the ROI or return on investment. They may not be aware that they ever had a breach or have never been subject to an investigation by a federal agency or OCR regarding health information security or privacy. Therefore, they continue to risk leaking sensitive information.

HOW WIDE ARE THE VARIATIONS?

Although information security efforts can land an organization of any type or size into difficulties, it is the smaller healthcare providers and their business associates who face the most struggles. The main reason why relatively few organizations have superior security programs in place is because it takes ongoing commitment and money from the levels of executives. Within an organization, program implementation may be uneven since a hospital may do some things professionally, but may lack in other areas.

Weaknesses in implementing these security measures are more prevalent in small clinics, physician practices and business associates. While some may be totally committed to privacy and security with their processes and cultures even so, a greater majority might be just starting to learn about how to implement measures to secure patient information. Such huge disparities are sadly not uncommon in the healthcare system.

However, under the HIPAA Omnibus Final Rule, business associates, similar to healthcare organizations, are liable for a direct compliance to HIPAA. Each violation of HIPAA by these vendors may land them OCR penalties to the tune of $1.5 million. Experts are finding that while many healthcare organizations are doing only average in their efforts, several business associates recently introduced to the compliance demands of HIPAA are unable to meet the requirements.

IS THERE ROOM FOR IMPROVEMENT?

Experts are of the view that the present situation of varying achievement among healthcare entities and business associates in their efforts towards information security is likely to continue for some time. However, those who struggle the most can improve their grades by following a few key steps.

OCR, in their pilot HIPAA compliance audit program conducted in 2012, evaluated 115 covered entities. They concluded that improvement requires following some basic steps, which they found were the major weaknesses.

The top priorities include conducting risk assessments, having procedures and policies in place and also encryption. OCR found that apart from these basic requirements in terms of kick starting a compliance program, an organization also needs to get a buy-in from its leaders, assign accountability as well as have a breach response protocol in place. Workforce awareness programs at most organizations need improvement, since breaches usually involve insiders.

For example, healthcare organizations typically adopt a volunteer firefighter model but do not take adequate steps to prepare for possible incidents. Instead they need to replace this with an advanced assignment of key players who would be involved with incident response. Although there are commercial training products available, most are inadequate with incorrect information about HIPAA and have poor test questions. Therefore, organizations intending to use such generic content must be sure to supplement or customize it with their own specific security policies.

David Holtzman, former senior advisor to the Office for Civil Rights (OCR), mentions a key factor that all business associates and healthcare entities must focus on when implementing information security programs. According to Holtzman, all data, including healthcare information, should be considered as the most important asset of the organization and appropriate steps taken to protect it. These steps must be on par with those taken to protect payment and financial streams that come through the organization. The entity must value its data just the same as it does any of its prime financial assets and invest in it.

HOW VULNERABLE IS THE HEALTHCARE SECTOR TO HACKERS?

L agging behind in addressing known problems, the healthcare industry remains one of the most vulnerable in the country.

Although the search for efficiency and improved care has taken the healthcare industry to the Internet in recent years, its medical devices and vulnerable hospital computers have been exposed to a wide variety of hacking in the process. According to security researchers, there are intruders waiting to exploit known gaps for stealing records of patients to then use them in identity theft schemes. They can even launch disruptive attacks to shut down critical hospital systems.

After conducting a one-year investigation on cyber-security, The Washington Post found that healthcare remains one of the most vulnerable sectors in the country, partly because of the delay in addressing known problems. The industry has a huge number of gaping security holes. If the financial industry were to handle security the way the healthcare industry is now, they would be stuffing cash in mattresses under their beds.

In comparison with the military, corporate and financial networks, hospitals and other medical facilities have faced relatively few hacks—that is, up until now. In the recent months, terrorists, criminals, cyber-warriors and activist hackers are finding healthcare an increasingly inviting target. Officials with the Department of Homeland Security confirm this. According to these sources, there is a growing tendency towards loss or theft of medical information and patient safety, because of these vulnerabilities.

When researched more deeply, according to The Washington Post, security experts find the same trivial-seeming flaws affecting the healthcare sector today as those that hackers exploited earlier to penetrate the computers at Google, the Pentagon and financial network services. The study also revealed that two major causes of persisting vulnerabilities within the healthcare industry are the routine failure to fix these known software flaws for ageing technology, and a culture of healthcare workers, nurses and physicians that do not follow basic measures of security such as not using passwords, in favor of convenience.

EXAMPLES OF TRIVIAL VULNERABILITIES

There were some disturbing findings revealed in The Washington Post investigation. A hospital in Oklahoma has a system that operates an electronic medicine cabinet. Weaknesses in the software interface allowed any unauthorized user to take it over easily.

The Peace Corps worldwide is about to adopt OpenEMR, a management system for electronic medical records. The software has several security flaws to allow hackers to break in easily.

A medical center at the University of Chicago has an unsecure Dropbox site so that new residents can use their iPads to manage patient care. They use a single user name and password, both of which they published in an online manual.

NOT KEEPING PACE WITH CHANGING TECHNOLOGY

Industry practices have not kept pace with the fast changing technology. Government oversight is partly to blame for this. Although the Food and Drug Administration is responsible for overseeing medical devices, their most recent guideline on cybersecurity was published back in 2005.

The agency does tell hospitals to seek help from vendors for guidance on security of sophisticated devices. Although the agency encourages such updates, vendors are often unable to update FDA-approved systems. That leaves those systems vulnerable to potential attacks and people are very confused about the position of FDA.

The Washington Post investigation also noted that although a report by the Government Accountability Office reported vulnerability of insulin pumps and defibrillators to hacks, a year later, one researcher-hacker used a specialized search engine and discovered a wireless glucose monitor in Wisconsin that was linked to the Internet and open to hacking.

The healthcare industry is moving toward electronic health records systems, overseen by the Department of Health and Human Services. However, there are documented security vulnerabilities in the system.

Although the HHS health information technology standards committee is of the view that the healthcare industry is working hard to overcome their shortcomings, other researchers are skeptical. They claim that several security flaws identified in electronic health record systems two years ago are yet to be rectified. That leaves the system open to exploitation by skilled hackers.

THE ONGOING CONCERN

For over a decade now, cybersecurity of medical systems has been under the lens. However, as hospitals are increasingly adopting the use of wireless systems and electronic records to manage patient data, the issue has magnified.

According to The Washington Post, the ICSA Labs that test for security products such as electronic health records for government certification, they do acknowledge healthcare systems rank near the bottom of the list. There are not many attacks, since typically attackers have been concentrating on money thus far. However, this finding should not make the industry complacent since identity theft is on the rise and patient information is sensitive to hacking. A faulty assumption among healthcare officials is that their networks offer too few financial enticements, or are too obscure to be of any interest to hackers.

THE ANECDOTES ARE MOUNTING

No one is exactly aware of how many intrusions occur at any given period. However, mounting anecdotes are causing concern. For example, during 2009 and 2011, malicious viruses infected medical devices at VA facilities at least 181 times. This was reported by DHS intelligence.

The Utah Health Department had their network server compromised, when a hacker gained access to Medicaid data belonging to 780,000 people and stole several of them. Computers in Eastern Europe were responsible and Utah officials say they have taken extensive measures to protect their patients.

THE STEP FORWARD

HHS has established an array of standards and to meet them, the law requires that independent labs certify electronic health records. However, the standards include only a few security provisions. The existing pattern of industry practices leaves commercial EHR systems vulnerable to exploitation, with only low skill levels sufficient to exploit them. Experts urge rigorous security testing before certifying vendors of electronic health records for stimulus funding. That makes it clear that federal certification standards are not sufficient.

A HEALTHCARE INDUSTRY ON IT LIFE SUPPORT

Controlling costs is paramount in any industry, but the healthcare industry is finding that safeguarding patient information in a digital world is not so easy.

WHY ARE MEDICAL RECORDS SO VULNERABLE?

The healthcare industry has lagged behind the rest of the corporate world in adapting integrated security systems. These are designed to prevent data from being moved into portable files. As a result, most healthcare organizations have sensitive data spread throughout various departments, providing plenty of opportunities for leaks.

In addition, the healthcare industry is extremely fragmented in nature. For example, there are several types of hospitals, a multitude of physicians, a large number of ambulatory healthcare providers and laboratories. In addition, there are the insurers and providers of collecting and billing services. The net result is that sensitive information is handled by several small and unsophisticated players, and they are not equipped with the correct tools to protect it.

The implications of the exposure of the health records of a person may not necessarily be limited to financial identity theft and or basic fraud. When the information ends up on the Internet, it may lead to social stigma and embarrassment for the patient. Criminals take advantage of the information by exploiting healthcare as well as stealing supplies and drugs. When a thief uses a stolen identity to gain medical care, the victim suffers because his medical records are corrupted by the medical data of the thief and it can carry adverse health consequences for the victim. Security experts have demonstrated how an insulin pump may be potentially hacked and used to deliver a lethal dose to an unsuspecting patient. Therefore, stopping fraud or even correcting it is a veritable nightmare for the industry.

REQUIRED TO BE PROACTIVE, NOT REACTIVE

Only a clear strategy and a strong blend of security measures can prevent such leakages. However, IT security in most healthcare industries is principally reactive and managers work to close the gaps only after the information has been leaked, or only to comply with the latest government regulation. As prevention is typically better than a cure, proactive investments invariably work better than investments made in security once the breach has occurred. Therefore, healthcare organizations can follow four steps for an effective approach to information security.

MONITOR—DATA FLOW

An inventory of the personal information and related sensitive data will reveal how it is being used in the organization, places where it is being stored and its route and passage as it flows through the organization and its partners. While doing so, security managers will uncover the weak spots where patient data is likely to be exposed improperly. Fortified with this knowledge, they can make an educated decision to identify and implement the proper security measures for reducing those risks.

ACCESS—CONTROL

This pertains to knowing who in the organization needs to see the personal data of a patient and under what circumstances. The healthcare industry has been historically built for openness rather than for security. Earlier, community media such as local newspapers and church bulletins would announce hospital admissions for encouraging volunteers to visit and help. Within the hospital, physical medical records were always on display so that any doctor or nurse could review a chart.

However, copying that openness into the electronic health record systems caused a lot of trouble, as openness and the digital world do not bond together. Here, sensitive data falling into wrong hands via network hacking, misdirected emails, stolen laptops and lost mobiles can cause untold damages.

One simple option is to limit the access to personal health information. However, that would have a devastating effect during an emergency. For example, other doctors may need immediate access to the data of a patient in an emergency, when his/her regular doctor is not available.

Just as firefighters have break-the-glass in case of emergencies, many hospitals and healthcare organizations also have systems in place that allow protected data to be accessed during medical crisis. However, that requires vigilance in weeding out cheaters from those who need to access it legitimately.

This has resulted in the development of a new type of access control system. It considers the identity of the person requesting the information while simultaneously considering the context of the request. For example, the UC Davis Health Systems uses an automated rolling audit of the emergency access for catching anomalies. Suspicious behavior, such as an employee accessing data of a patient with the same last name (posing as a relative), is flagged and leads to investigations and further manual audits.

EASY-TO-USE-TECHNOLOGY

When IT installs a security application that is difficult for people to use, it causes bigger problems. For example, a virtual private network was installed in a hospital for ensuring a secure connection to patient data when doctors would work from home. However, the network was so slow that doctors found it easier to export data into files and send it to their personal email accounts. This resulted in a much bigger problem compared to the original.

Typically, when an application does not work as intended or is too difficult to use in practice, people resort to various workarounds, fuelling data hemorrhages. Frustration leads users to move data into formats such as Excel and Word, which are more convenient but infinitely less secure. In the process of making data more portable, it becomes vulnerable.

EDUCATION—FOR EMPLOYEES AND DOCTORS

Most doctors consider themselves as the ultimate arbiter of happenings within their sphere of influence. That presents a peculiar challenge in this area. Traditional security education such as messages that scare users into changing their passwords periodically, does not typically work on this audience.

Doctors also prefer not to carry more than one device. In other fields such as investment banking, it is common to find professionals carrying multiple handheld devices such as a Blackberry for protecting sensitive data, and another phone for personal use. Healthcare practitioners show a preference for consumer devices such as iPads as their technology of choice. In an ever evolving industry, software is available that provides security for business applications on phones and tablets, while allowing users to enjoy social media and games.

However, not every problem can be solved simply by technology alone. The key lies in educating healthcare professionals that security hygiene is just as important as any other risk in caring for a patient. This is what it ultimately boils down to—caring for the patient—something that all in the healthcare industry are passionate about.

ASSESSING HEALTHCARE INFOSEC COMPETENCY

Professional credentialing is often required for substantiation of information security and privacy work in healthcare environments.

THE SITUATION IN THE HEALTHCARE INDUSTRY

For the most part, the healthcare industry is comprised of junior staff. Although these people may have grown with and have different roles within the organization, protecting electronic assets or handling electronic information is a brand new responsibility for them. The compliance officer, CISO or the CIO needs something tangible when assessing a person to decide whether he/she has what it takes to address the complex needs of privacy and information security in a healthcare environment.

The healthcare industry needs to be able to nurture their personnel in such a manner that they will give it a tangible return on investment. This must be clearly visible and the level of competency obtained must be quantifiable and measurable by an authorized third party. For example, many areas of information security are automated, such as with remote software patching. The healthcare environment, however, has special purpose computing platforms and advanced medical devices that are typically not served with automation.

Medical staff has to accommodate the equipment and understand that a lot of it must be updated and upgraded manually. It requires coordination with the manufacturers of these medical devices to make sure they have tested the patch and approved it. Consequently, personnel in the healthcare workforce need to be aware of the complexity and should be able to work through these processes. Ongoing training must be provided so that the personnel is properly equipped to manage such sensitive material.

The changing demands of healthcare privacy and security work require measuring the competency of the individuals. The (ISC)2 or the International Information System Security Certification Consortium offers the HealthCare Information Security and Privacy Practitioners. (HCISPP) credential. This requires the individual to maintain the level of education annually, while staying current in the profession. It also requires them to grow and evolve as a privacy and security professional in the healthcare information security environment.

INFOSEC QUALIFICATION FOR HEALTHCARE

The new certification, HCISPP, offered by (ISC)2, is the first foundational global standard that assesses both information privacy and security expertise within the healthcare industry. The credential is available worldwide, and the body says it is designed to provide both the healthcare employers and the people in the industry with substantiation suitable for a practitioner of healthcare privacy and security. It provides the assurance that the healthcare privacy and security practitioner has the essential level of expertise and knowledge required by the industry for addressing specific concerns of info-security.

In keeping with the standard of its other credentials, (ISC)2 had to conduct a JTA or job task analysis study for determining the scope and content of the HCISPP. Industry luminaires from the US, Hong Kong and Europe, including subject matter experts from other (ISC) membership attended several workshops for exam development and contributed towards developing the CBK or common body of knowledge that now serves as the foundation for the credential.

HCISPP requires applicants to have at least two years of experience in the single knowledge area of the credential that includes privacy, compliance and security. Applicants with legal experience may use it to substitute for compliance and those with experience in information management may substitute it for privacy. Of the two years of experience, one of them must be in the healthcare industry. In order to achieve the HCISPP credentials, all candidates must demonstrate their competencies in the following six CBK domains:

- Information governance and risk management
- Security and privacy in healthcare
- Regulatory Environment
- Third party risk management
- Information risk assessment
- Healthcare Industry

HCISPP differentiates itself from other certifications in several ways. The primary difference is its international scope which benefits both employers as well as individuals. This is crucial in adopting and driving practices for properly storing, securing and exchanging sensitive healthcare data.

The (ISC)2 credential takes great care to provide assurance that a candidate has a comprehensive understanding of HIPAA's requirements for not only the US and Europe, but also those of other places that have extremely strict requirements regarding the protection of personal data, its sharing, and actions to be taken in the event of a breach.

Although a candidate may obtain a HIPAA awareness certificate by attending a training class and passing an exam, the new HCISPP credential is much more comprehensive and all encompassing. It is designed such that it can critically assess the understanding of an individual in implementing, managing and accessing privacy and security controls, which require experience and complete comprehension of how to apply that knowledge to the healthcare environment.

WHO SHOULD CONSIDER OBTAINING CERTIFICATION?

According to (ISC)2, those considering obtaining the new certification would include security and privacy consultants, health information managers, IT managers, medical records supervisors, risk analysis, compliance auditors, information security officers, compliance officers and privacy officers.

WHO MIGHT CONSIDER HIRING THOSE WITH THE CREDENTIAL?

According to (ISC)2, employers who might be interested in hiring those who have earned the HCISPP credential would include regulatory agencies, claims processors, consulting firms, physician group practices and hospitals. They might also encourage existing personnel to obtain the credential.

As the HIPAA Omnibus Rule requires business associates of the healthcare industry to comply with HIPAA also, these vendors may also consider that their staff members attain the credential. Alternately, business associate staff may find merit in a healthcare specific certification if they do not have any credentials today.

However, earning the right security certification does not make it a one-size-fits-all solution. It depends on the individual, their intended career path and their current role in their industry. Some may be looking for a broad knowledge base, while others might be searching for something specific that can support technical skills such as architecture or networking.

HOW HEALTHCARE PROVIDERS CAN ASSESS THEIR RISKS

Healthcare organizations need a robust risk assessment methodology, wherein they can protect their patient data, comply with regulations as well as support other business initiatives.

With the inception of HIPAA in 1996, it became necessary for healthcare organizations to implement a risk methodology for accurately identifying and mitigating risks within their environment. This risk methodology forms a foundational IT security process, which is essential when making educated decisions about protocol. Although several healthcare organizations do start the process for risk methodology adoption, there are many that face different drawbacks and delays.

QUALITATIVE OR QUANTITATIVE

Often, organizations do not consider what type of risk methodology they should adopt. They may go along with whatever is the current Hot Topic methodology, such as the NIST SP 800-30, without giving much thought to, or even understanding the purpose of the methodology and how to implement it appropriately. Although risk methodologies can be considered as best practices,

cessarily be a good fit for every organization. Imple-
ive or observed approaches may be easier to imple-
o not use factual data when determining risk. On
other nand, implementing quantitative or scientific approaches
may be difficult, requiring a significant amount of ongoing effort,
but these provide more thorough and accurate results.

Whatever methodology an organization may choose to implement,
some common actions are necessary to be implemented:

- Identifying all devices in the organizations

- An understanding of all the inputs, outputs, and flow of data

- Identifying the threats and vulnerabilities associated with
  each device

- Identifying the threat tolerance of the organization, and the
  level of uncertainty for each device

Organizations usually have several departments with varying priorities existing in a diverse and constantly changing environment.
The above actions must be completed with the information available from each and every department.

COMPARING APPLES TO ORANGES

Popular risk methodologies typically do not include factors outside of information security. While information security happens
to be only one piece of the jigsaw puzzle it does not mean that
information security risk is comparable to operational, compliance
or financial risks, since comparing them is like comparing apples
to oranges. The entire organization cannot take advantage of the
same risk methodology, since the goal is to define individual critical organizational factors, such as operational, compliance, financial and information security, all distilling into an overall organizational risk methodology.

Such a holistic approach will give rise to actionable results for business, in turn resulting in the business addressing risks, providing support, and allocating the necessary funds for information security.

MANAGEMENT OF EXCEPTIONS

The risk assessment methodology adopted by organizations may have an exception process included within them. However, in most cases, the person accepting the risk is typically not provided with adequate information to make an educated decision. Administration will often willingly approve an exception, if it results in business goals being achieved sooner, regardless of the effectiveness of any control for mitigation. For example, in the absence of proper cross-functional education, the owner of a business may not understand Cross Site Request Forgery, its impact on their application, or the organization, or the necessity for it to be remediated before an application is promoted to production.

Additionally, exceptions must never be made permanent. Most organizations typically do not review exceptions regularly as a process, nor verify if they are still valid or presenting the same level of impact and likelihood as when they were initially identified.

EXCLUSION OF EXECUTIVE LEADERSHIP

Operations management commonly handles information security risks. Managers making decisions for mitigating risks do not always have the authority to hire additional resources, allocate additional budget or influence priorities across departments. Resource constraints together with absence of C-level support and decision making can often defer changes required for mitigating risks on to the ten-year road map of the organization.

NARROW FOCUS

Many organizations, especially those small and medium sized, depend solely on external sources as methods of identifying risk. For example, organizations typically use new releases from a vendor patch subscription for identifying their risk. Some use the results of an application scanning for vulnerabilities. However, depending solely on external sources does not take into consideration other factors such as internal/external audits, legacy systems, changes in business processes, new systems, new business relationships, changing compliance requirements or new technology.

AREAS TO CONSIDER

Organizations starting a risk assessment must consider the following areas:

- Do not attempt to implement a best practice risk methodology without first determining if it is the best fit for your organization

- Do not define or execute the risk methodology without adequate inputs and support

- Do not exclude the risk factors from outside of information security

- Do your research for determining the methodology that will support the organization in the best possible way

- Do risk assessments regularly

- Do form a risk management committee that will discuss risks, make a determination on risk ratings and approve exceptions

HEALTHCARE SECURITY CHALLENGES AND TRAINING

Although there are several obstacles in healthcare, providers want to be familiar with some of the new-age best practices.

Data breaches due to human error have not slowed down the healthcare industry, despite new social engineering attacks continuing to be on the rise. Users in healthcare organizations regularly face various pitfalls such as phishing schemes, and privacy and security officers need to be constantly aware of these threats.

The healthcare industry is increasingly adopting new technology and filtering massive amounts of data through them. That means there is no single set of policies or products that can help users in these organizations adhere to the best practices of security. Rather, providers need to seek out newer technologies available for determining what best fits their organization.

CHALLENGES IN SECURING PATIENT DATA

The rapid increase in different types of mobile devices present the main challenge for securing patient data. Apart from such mobile devices requiring physical security, they also need protection from spyware/malware that could easily penetrate the device.

User training is the next big challenge. Users who update and share confidential patient information need training about the best practices to be followed. The challenge is that training is not always consistent for all users. For instance, data security and best practices training required by a front desk person will be different from that required by a coder (ICD-10) or a Physician. Personalizing training materials based on the user being trained, although a challenging prospect in itself, would no doubt help in users accepting them more readily.

Simple PowerPoint presentations no longer cut it. Proper training must be done over time, with plenty of repetition and feedback from the user. For example, the Drayer Physical Therapy Institute relies on Security Awareness Training KnowBe4 to help them stay on top of current threats and potential social attacks.

TECHNOLOGIES SUITABLE FOR PRIVACY AND SECURITY IN ORGANIZATIONS

Information present on digital storage media must be encrypted with any one of the suitable technologies available, such as PGP or Pretty Good Privacy. That will make the data useless to any unauthorized person, and in the event of a breach, the information stays intact. While sharing, users need to send encrypted data via secured communications networks using technologies such as SSH to reduce the risk of data breaches.

Within the organization, security of data may be ensured with Access Control technologies, such as strong passwords and biometrics (finger print scanners). With proper access control implementation, users are granted permission only for what they need and are allowed to perform only those tasks in the system that have been pre selected for them, based on their position.

Cloud computing systems can help the organization to consolidate data, and over time, the operation is less expensive. However, compliance issues must be taken into account including latory challenges for making a smooth transition.

Vendors play a major role in deciding the technology most suitable for an organization. As every organization is different, it can decide the security it wants on top of the vendor product and the vendor might help in the integration. Another way this can work is by the vendor pro-actively integrating the latest in security offerings onto their product. Either way, vendors need to consider agile processes seriously, because security updates need to be presented to the customer frequently for minimizing risk.

WHAT SHOULD BE THE FOCUS IN TRAINING?

Although there will be gaps in the security culture of any organization, including gaps within their policies, procedures and infrastructure, it is more imperative to plug the gaps in people's behavior. Just as a driver on the road has a social responsibility to be safe, users must be willing to take on the responsibility for security.

That requires a security awareness program. In this area, policies and procedures are not really effective unless users are aware of the security risks they are taking when they click without thinking.

Effective user training is required so that users are able to spot the problems as quickly as possible. Using cloud solutions such as KnowBe4 may be suitable, as it does not tax the present infrastructure.

The training must begin with new hires with an onboarding training process. They start with policy descriptions and expectations and move on to practical sessions on in-house phishing scams so that they are ready for threats from the real world. With organizations using BYOD more often, operating systems on the devices will need anti-virus and anti-malware protection. Users need to be made aware of these protection schemes, as nearly 99% do not have any protection in their devices.

Training must be effective if users are expected to handle sophisticated attacks. Simply dumping training data on users does not work anymore. Designated training sessions and manuals should be mandatory. Training should make users think twice before they click on something. While at the work place, they need to adopt a different way of thinking which includes a change to—"How is this sender sending me a personal email when they should not have my work email address?" It is extremely important to ensure the effectiveness of training with suitable metrics.

COMMON USER PATTERNS DETECTED DURING TRAINING

Most user executives may not want their employees to take time out for training on security awareness. It is important for the organization to realize that if their system becomes compromised, it would take up even more of their employees' time, additional resources and possibly tarnish their brand.

CYBERDRILL, THREATS AND HEALTHCARE CYBERSECURITY

Apart from the need to improve willingness to share cyber-security information, many healthcare organizations must also be willing to improve their basic cyber-security defenses.

A cyber-security drill conducted by the HHS or the Health and Human Services together with HITRUST or the Health Information Trust Alliance on April 1, 2014 resulted in findings that healthcare organizations should target improving their basic mechanism of defense against cyber-attacks. Simultaneously, they should also improve their willingness to share information regarding cyber threats. They have also studied the emerging threats facing the healthcare industry and the ongoing efforts towards its security by HealthCare.gov.

CHALLENGES FACING THE HEALTHCARE SECTOR

The drill found that the healthcare ecosystem is no different from other sectors as far as the challenges it faces compared to what others do; the threats are common—hacktivism, state-sponsored threats, bad behavior from employees and organized crime—both intentional and unintentional. However, the difference where the healthcare sector stands out is that there exists a huge resistance towards implementation of best practices of information security, this being an additional challenge for the industry sector. Most often, on one hand, organizations are not willing to share information regarding their security breaches and incidents of cyber-crime. On the other, clinicians shun technologies such as multi-factor authentication.

A PEEK INTO THE CYBERRX DRILL

Information security teams conducted the recent CyberRX drill at several hospitals and health insurance companies, healthcare providers, a large nationwide retail pharmacy chain and 13 unnamed healthcare sector companies. Of the four exercises conducted, two involved a compromised medical device and ran for over a seven-hour period. They also included a simulated attack on a state health insurance exchange that was connected to the federally facilitated insurance marketplace belonging to HealthCare.gov of the HHS.

Compared with others, the healthcare sector has an added risk. This sector is a complex web of hundreds of thousands of providers and a massive conglomerate of interconnected systems, devices, the government and acts such as the Affordable Care Act. According to the first set of exercises, the primary challenge in the healthcare sector is the concern of liability leading to reluctance in sharing information about attacks and threats with the rest of the sector.

As such the concern of liability is from a company standpoint, rather than from the cyber-security side. It boils down to the liability introduced into the company environment when information about a breach or other problems is shared. Healthcare organizations are concerned about what they share and how so that it does not cause them any liability.

This concern about liability is at the root of why there is not much sharing between industries, despite the executive orders from

President Obama. The order encourages sharing between the private sectors, public sectors, and the federal government in order to improve cyber-security and situational awareness, while improving overall security.

Along with the reluctance to share information about cyber-threats, attacks and incidents, the first drill also indicated that many healthcare entities must still iron out their defense mechanisms. Basically, some participating organizations find that they have yet to set up proper processes and methods when dealing with an incident. This involves fundamentals such as basically knowing whom to call when an incident does occur.

Among the pool of participants, some organizations had mature programs, which they exercised, but several others did not, and realized the gaps. The next exercise to be conducted later in the year will have a larger sample size, which will enable examination of why some organizations are better prepared than others.

The drills have evoked a good response from more than 300 healthcare related organizations. This is especially so because the participants undergoing that drill found an opportunity to exercise their internal processes for incident response and ways to improve.

RESISTANCE TO BEST PRACTICES

Another finding of the drill is that the healthcare sector resists implementation of best practices as a whole, for information security. For example, physicians demonstrate a lot of resistance to the use of two-factor authentication.

Conducting drills such as CyberRX, together with education and communication, helps to make people understand the actual and real risks involved with such threats. Although there has been a lot of fear mongering, to date, HealthCare.gov has not faced any successful malicious attacks on their systems or on their site. Additionally, HealthCare.gov is currently undergoing comprehensive security testing every three months, even though the federal government has a guideline, such rigorous testing take place every three years.

HealthCare.gov is likely to continue being tested every quarter for another year or two, before a reasonable cycle is decided. As insurers offer new health plans, the security team and HealthCare.gov will be busy updating the site and systems, with the process being a continual improvement for the site.

The healthcare sector is no different from other industries when it comes to emerging cyber-threats. Those include organized crime circles and threats posed by insiders involving theft of data to commit fraud. However, the healthcare sector faces additional threats from nation-states as well, where the focus of that threat is on stealing intellectual property.

The US healthcare sector has the best technologies, devices, software, drugs and electronic medical records under development. Nation states are mostly interested in IP, because they would not need to conduct their own research if they can steal from someone else.

PREVENTING HEALTHCARE ORGANIZATION FRAUD INVOLVING INSIDERS

Healthcare organizations need to stay vigilant in restricting staff access to patient information and ramp up employee training.

Recently three incidents of identity theft have highlighted that healthcare organizations need to stay watchful, and prevent fraud involving insiders. These are the incidents:

- Seven individuals arrested in Louisiana had among them a former hospital-billing worker. He was allegedly using patient information and creating fake checks and IDs.

- A former hospital emergency department clerk in Florida accessed above 750,000 patient records and sold the information for profit.

- A former state employee of Texas used patient immunization records and applied online for credit cards.

According to security experts, healthcare organizations need to take several steps for minimizing the risk of identity theft. Apart from monitoring worker activity and auditing them, they must restrict staff access to information of patients and ramp up training for employees.

THE LOUISIANA CASE

The billing worker used copies of scanned checks from a database and other patient information at the LSU Hospital System and created fake IDs and checks to be used by others. So far, more than 400 patients from several states are said to have been affected, although the number may go up as LSU and the state police continue to investigate the matter further.

All policies and procedures of the organization are under review in the wake of the incident and new procedures are under formulation, to be put into effect very soon. According to a State Police spokesman, although ID thefts are nothing new, this case is different because several individuals were involved and a large amount of information was taken out from the hospital database, which is unusual in cases involving counterfeit checks.

THE FLORIDA CASE

An emergency department registration worker and his wife, an insurance representative, both working for the Florida Hospital Celebration, conspired to obtain health information. The former clerk used a computer in his department and accessed electronic health records inappropriately to collect data on more than 750,000 patients from several Florida Hospital locations.

He selected information on individuals involved in motor vehicle accidents to solicit them for chiropractic and legal services. The clerk sold the collected patient information to a third person for profit.

THE TEXAS CASE

It is not just hospitals that are vulnerable to such insider ID thefts. More than a hundred individuals had their information stolen from the Texas Department of Health and Human Services, when a former worker used their information from immunization records. He used the stolen data to apply online for credit cards.

The information stolen included names of the family members of the patient and their Social Security numbers.

According to a recent survey, it is relatively common to find cases of medical identity theft. The survey, conducted by the Ponemon Institute, a research firm, involved 80 healthcare organizations. They found that more than 50 percent had one or multiple incidents of medical identity thefts over the past one year, while only one third had sufficient controls in place for detecting medical identity thefts.

STEPS HEALTHCARE ORGANIZATIONS CAN TAKE FOR FRAUD PREVENTION

For preventing ID theft, one of the most important steps that healthcare organizations can take is to monitor the computer activity of their employees regularly. This will allow detection of inappropriate or unusual access, printing of patient information and transmission of data.

As suggested by David Harlow, founder of The Harlow Group LLC consulting firm, healthcare should follow the lead of the financial services industry. Employees must take a mandatory two weeks annual vacation, so that the organization can audit the worker's activities during his time off.

According to David, clinics, hospitals and others should limit patient information access based on job duties. Information could be divided up such that no one person has access to all the information that he might use for fraud. For instance, Social Security numbers should not be accessible to employees in the billing department.

ROLE BASED ACCESS

Configuring the storage systems for enforcing role-based access to information can actually boost compliance to HIPAA. For example, a worker with the ER admissions does not need access to information related to patient treatment. The hospital must insist that the third-party software it uses has such controls baked into it.

Unfortunately, healthcare organizations often do not tap such capabilities even if the technology is available to them for controlling employee access to patient data. For example, even when role-based access to patient data is employed, many hospitals do not take the time to fine-tune the granularity of the control.

Finally, as a critical deterrent to ID theft, healthcare organizations must place special emphasis on employee training and re-training, with special highlights on the rules and regulations, including the consequences and penalties of illegal or inappropriate activity.

HOW IS THE OZONE FRAMEWORK EXPECTED TO REVOLUTIONIZE THE HEALTHCARE INDUSTRY?

A mandate by the National Defense Authorization Act 2012 has declared the NSA project Ozone Widget Framework as open source.

THE OZONE WIDGET FRAMEWORK

The US Congress, along with the Department of Defense has recognized that OWF or the Ozone Widget Framework software helps effectively in the development and support of mission-critical applications. Originally, OWF was created as a platform for military command centers and used for web-based analytics. Today, health and disease management systems are using OWF increasingly.

OWF is a web application and it is open-source. As it is highly customizable, it assembles the tools required for accomplishing any task automatically, allowing the tools to communicate among themselves. The application is a framework permitting developers to select from a library of widgets that can perform specific functions for exchanging information; no special programming skills are required.

Widgets are a familiar feature thanks to their prolific use in tablets and smartphones. The most common example is Google MAPS and Voice Search is another. As developers are able to use OWF, through customization, they extend the layers for specific use. Anyone can extend or modify the code, since the software is open-source.

Using a dashboard, developers can easily select required widgets to build an application, which then acts as a web-portal for displaying the selected widgets in separate frames. Data exchange between different widgets happens in real time. According to NSA, OWF is under testing by the Army and the Navy internally, for creating a marketplace. Here, users can easily find and download applications. Using an Ozone software development kit, outside developers can write and publish their apps to the marketplace.

The key benefit form OWF comes in the form of rapid prototyping and integration of operational data and real-time intelligence. Since a widget is a visual component positioned on a board, the Table Widget provides visual representations of tabular data in a familiar tabular format. There can be one or more widgets individually displaying a section of the data for visualization.

For example, AppBoard has one or more widgets and presents the data objects visually, while running in the Flash Virtual Machine. There is no restriction on the display and it can contain any type of widget. That allows the system designer to present the data objects in the most suitable format that is of the utmost value to the end-user. Widgets may typically be of the type:

- Graph or Chart
- Table or Data Grid
- Topological Map for representing the structure of a network
- Geographical Map for displaying data overlaid on a map

THE OZONE WIDGET FRAMEWORK IN HEALTH INFORMATION SYSTEMS

Typically, problems with Big Data means the inability to analyze large volumes in real time as rapidly increasing information is collected across disparate systems. That additionally means no communication of the analysis exists across different types of users.

In the past, systems collected data and processed them in information silos, while analysts used separate applications and output formats. The method was time consuming and at best, it was a past-view model of the situation. Since the Internet is now a dominant means for data sharing, applications use XML and similar standards for interpreting and communicating different data types. File based data, after morphing from database platforms to relational databases, is currently moving towards columnar-based systems.

Big Data problems are further compounded by the explosion of devices connecting through IP addresses rather than via people. For example, the Internet of Things is transforming data analytics in several innovative ways:

- Genomists in the area of disease and health information are using different systems for accumulating and exchanging scientific data. By adopting the OWF platform, they can use a single metadata repository for connecting and analyzing information through a single portal.

- European CDC is testing epidemic intelligence using OWF for monitoring health data collected from various networks and several medical facilities.

- Emerging countries are expanding telemedicine healthcare along with smartphone apps taking advantage of cellular communication, since that provides a cost effective way to capture, analyze and share patient data.

- OWF, slated to operate on smartphones and tablets in the future, can help doctors in serology, diagnosis of diseases and data collection via CAT, PET and X-ray images.

- OWF applications are finding growth markets in implant devices with remote monitoring features. Diabetes control, pulmonary edema monitoring, heart pacemakers and implants for detecting the onset of seizures can create substantial data flows that a standard set of widgets can display for analysis. Since OWF is capable of supporting data captured from sensors in the field, it can support similar requirement in health monitoring.

CONCLUSION:

OWF is not unique, since the market place has several web portal information systems. However, it is valuable as it is open source, reflecting significant investments from the US taxpayers and it can now be applied to solving healthcare information stranded with Big Data problems. The challenge will come from the for-profit healthcare providers—whether they will be willing to adhere to a common platform for information exchange and data analysts across the chain of healthcare providers, insurers and public agencies.

NETWORK SECURITY'S EFFECT ON WIRELESS UPGRADES

From a network perspective, security is increasingly becoming an important factor, since healthcare organizations have a lot of clinical devices on the network, which are vulnerable to attackers.

Healthcare institutions extensively use wireless technology in a wide variety of settings. The emergency room, the pediatric ward, the intensive care unit and other departments all need Wi-Fi coverage, with each area requiring different considerations.

BENEFITS AND CHALLENGES OF WIRELESS NETWORKING IN HEALTHCARE

The most significant benefit of having a wireless network in a medical institution is that providers are able to deploy technology at the bedside of patients as a part of normal healthcare workflow. For example, smartphones access clinical data, while biomedical devices record and manage patient information. According to researchers, by 2014, wireless medical devices will be monitoring about 6 million patients.

Medical radio frequency identification or RFID technology keeps track of medical equipment throughout a hospital. Allowing visitors and patients to use Wi-Fi during hospital visits, boosts their satisfaction.

However, there are big challenges when healthcare units go wireless. Life-saving devices need a high-availability network for support. The network must also support movement of large amounts of data as required by electronic health records or EHR systems.

Wireless networking faces infrastructure issues such as rooms with lead-lined walls and old buildings with thick walls. It must also serve a varied user base that is highly mobile, including patients, guests, doctors and clinical staff. Any healthcare organization that supports a wireless network must consider the privacy and security regulations related to sensitive patient information.

REQUIREMENTS FOR A NEW WIRELESS INFRASTRUCTURE

Since new devices will be connecting to its network as its wireless infrastructure expands, the healthcare organization must ensure that patient data remain secure. This was the major requirement for Torrance Memorial Medical Center, which wanted to improve its wireless infrastructure in its existing hospital building, adjacent facilities, and its upcoming new medical tower.

Torrance is a non-profit medical center in Los Angeles County. It has 401 beds, 900 physicians and 3,500 employees on staff. Treating 23,000 patients annually, the healthcare organization has a large volunteer population and has to account for the huge volume of wireless and mobile devices connected to its network. Torrance announced that it was deploying a wireless LAN or Local Area Network from Aruba.

At high level, Torrance is concerned about two major areas in security. There is a guest network used by patients and visitors while they are in the hospital. This needs to remain separate from the networks used by the employees and clinical staff. Therefore, separation between the two networks is an important factor to the hospital, for which, they use ClearPass and AirWave for effective network management. While expanding, they hope to use these two technology platforms along with mobile device management or MDM.

THE OVERALL CHALLENGE

Although Torrance is currently implementing an MDM solution, the overall challenge is in letting users access the network with their mobile devices for their emails. For example, it is mandatory for users to change their passwords every 90 days. On failing to do so, their wireless devices will lock out their accounts. Moreover, it is important to ensure that all mobile devices used are secure, as Torrance has several clinical devices on the network.

Medical devices on the network may have vulnerabilities and different vulnerabilities of various types of devices, including medical devices, are listed on web sites. Therefore, security is becoming increasingly important from the perspective of a network. Threats such as Distributed Denial of Service are common and hackers scan the networks frequently, trying to take advantage of a connected device and its vulnerability.

Torrance has a partner for SIEM or Security Incident and Event Manager, to whom it sends its logs. Occasionally, the partner finds a wireless device is in communication with a bad IP on the internet. Usually, there are a few instances in a week, and this is a typical sign of an active malware on the device. Once the device is detected, ClearPass and Airwave identify the device its IP, and the IP it connects to, for determining what the problem is.

As more and more devices need to go onto an organization's networks, the challenge is to connect them to the network, while ensuring the devices are not being used for sharing patient information and that the network remains compliant.

THE WIRELESS INFRASTRUCTURE AND POLICIES

Torrance was seeking a solution that would allow users to connect their mobile devices, while the network remained HIPAA compliant. The solution they found most suitable was to set up a firewall that defines the reach of each user on the network, whenever they connect. Using their wireless infrastructure and ClearPass for policies, Torrance defined access based on device or role, and from where they were connecting. For example, a physician entering the network using a hospital-issued device can only have access to one part of the network.

PLANNING FOR A HEALTHCARE WIRELESS NETWORK

Proper planning is the key to the present and future needs of a hospital wireless network implementation. A good understanding of the habits of the current users helps decide the physical environment where the Wi-Fi is to be installed. Such planning may require hiring a consultant.

Experts are of the opinion that proper planning of a wireless network in a hospital requires thinking and planning ahead for the future—new technologies will invariably need the support of extra bandwidth. As care delivery enters new paradigms, the development of a wireless infrastructure within a hospital may require handling of highly mobile patients, healthcare data flow to several devices simultaneously in various locations, decentralized nurses, and many more.

LAUNCHING THE CLINICAL QUALITY FRAMEWORK & HEALTH EDECISION INITIATIVE CLOSE-OUT

Increasing efficiency while improving health and healthcare is paramount and for that the key parts are measuring and improving quality.

Within the S&I or Standards Interoperability framework, the HeD or Health eDecisions project has been leading the charge in accelerating standards for supporting the clinical decision support.

Although the HeD initiative came to a close on March 27, it is only the beginning of their quality efforts and not the end. A new initiative, the CQF or Clinical Quality Framework has been launched in collaboration with CMS or Centers for Medicare and Medicaid Services.

This new collaborative initiative, CQF, will use the work done by the HeD project as its foundation, and will be focusing on harmonizing the standards for electronic clinical quality measurement and clinical decision support. The HeD initiative has already done incredible work for the standards community, and some of their significant achievements are highlighted here.

ACHIEVEMENTS OF THE HED INITIATIVE

Launched in June 2012, the Health eDecision Initiative was handled by a dedicated, passionate and well-organized community. It achieved significant progress in harmonizing standards for CDS or Clinical Decision Support. It took the HeD community less than two years for completing work on two Use Cases:

CDS Artifact Sharing—This Use Case solved the dilemma of sharing a good clinical decision support rule with others via an electronic format, such that they are able to use the rule in their electronic health record.

CDS Guidance Service—This Use Case solved the technical difficulty of sending important data to an up to date service or website that provides advice on immunizations or other decisions of complex nature.

Although it sounds simple enough, this work was no small feat considering how difficult it is to develop standards or the challenges to be faced to get national consensus on standards. Not only did the HeD community evaluate and harmonize standards for Clinical Decision Support, they authored six HL7 standards with the help of the HL7 Work Group of the CDS and created three implementation guides. HL7 is ready to use and test all the standards and implementation guides as "draft standards". Among these standards are the:

- Implementation Guide for Clinical Decision Support knowledge Artifact
- Implementation Guide for Decision Support Service
- Standard for DSS or Decision Support Service
- Templates for vMR or Virtual Medical Record
- Specification for vMR XML
- Logical Model for vMR

The two Implementation Guides have already been included in the proposed notice published in the Federal Register, as appearing in the 2015 Edition NPRM. The HeD team also coordinated pilots of both the Use Cases with various vendors and content providers. After this, they also held the first ever Virtual Open House for S&I Pilots.

Clinical Decision Support is the representation of clinical guidance facing the user. For effective intervention of CDS, it is necessary that there is person-specific data, availability of computable biomedical knowledge and an inference or reasoning mechanism to combine these elements for generating and presenting actionable and helpful information to individuals, clinicians or caregivers in the proper way and at the proper time.

So that these benefits can be optimized, CDS interventions must be more easily implementable and shareable, such that any organization can easily acquire and deploy the interventions. For this, advanced standards are necessary to enable either the regular or the routine consumption of CDS intervention via a web service or by repeatedly importing and updating the CDS artifacts into CDS systems.

Another first, the Virtual Closing Ceremony of the S&I Initiative on March 27 honored those who participated in the initiative as an appreciation for all the hard work done by the community. The virtual closing ceremony included a review of the accomplishments of the initiative, insights from the participants of the HeD initiative and shared the "real world" applications of their work.

STAYING AHEAD OF THE SECURITY CURVE IN A COMMUNITY HOSPITAL

A smaller community hospital usually lacks the same level of funding and resources that are available in a larger healthcare network or hospital. Therefore, it is forced to maximize what it already has in place to stay in line with federal regulations. The type of security work and privacy required of community hospitals in many ways can be compared to that of a small-market sports team competing against a national team that has all the resources.

Typically, community hospitals, for example the Lawrence General Hospital, have to deal with the realities of information breaches and potential federal audits on a moderately restricted IT security budget. Throughout the US, there are thousands of such community hospitals, and they all face the same or similar challenges. Being the custodians of their patients' data, every CIO of these community hospitals has to focus primarily on the privacy and security of PHI. However, Lawrence General has been somewhat more innovative on the program side, and has filled some of those gaps.

As Lawrence General does not have a formal CISO or Chief Information Security Officer, its CIO serves as the de facto CISO, although there is a separate Privacy Officer who is also a domain expert. In other smaller community hospitals also, this is a fairly common practice, but Lawrence General has a robust Information Security or IS program that sets it apart for other similar organizations. However, the team at Lawrence General has to maintain equilibrium when building a secure infrastructure, while simultaneously working with new technological products.

Since it is not a large academic medical center, Lawrence General has to be prudent in whatever investments it makes. One of the biggest challenges they have to tackle is security, which they feel is expanding by the week. To "keep an eye on the ball", they need to handle this from a fiscal, resource and procedure/policy perspective for ensuring that they remain in line with and can monitor the latest security regulations and protocols continuously, on the state and federal level. In some ways, this proves to be an advantage for them, since not having the same funding or resources of a larger academic medical center, Lawrence General is forced to be more nimble and focused.

The community hospital augments the IS program with the help of an outside security consulting team for yearly assessments of its risk and security arrangements. For example, the consulting team has many widgets in the hospital's data center set to monitor its firewalls and data at rest behind the scenes. Whenever the hospital finds anything that is even remotely suspicious, it engages the same security team on a retainer. Dedicated security experts then determine whether it is a virus or something more sinister. According to the IS team of Lawrence General, these incidents are treated as great learning opportunities for the organization.

Lawrence General's concern with the audit side extends to continually making sure that in the event of an audit occurring, not only will they be compliant with the standard procedures and protocols that the HHS or Department of Health and Human Services would be looking for, but they are able to carry it a step further. Apart from looking at HIPAA Privacy and Security Rules, they are also targeting things such as NIST and DoD or Department or Defense level standards and protocols.

Within their IS program, Lawrence General has created a tiered matrix consisting of HIPAA, NIST and the DoD. That means stretching the IS team just a bit more than the basics. Although their line of action is no secret, they prefer to avoid the state of many hospitals that are in the practice of getting their yearly security audit, which finally turns into a piece of paper adorning a shelf. Lawrence General understands that over the last few years, compliance has evolved to a point where it has to be given its due importance as a program and that the piece of paper must be constantly reviewed and kept updated.

HOW CATHOLIC HEALTH SYSTEM BOOSTS THEIR NETWORK AND DATA CENTER SECURITY

Supporting BYOD, implementing PAC apps and EMR can be a significant challenge for healthcare industries with aging legacy networks.

THE CHALLENGE

Modern data centers, especially in healthcare industries, must cope with a vast range of security challenges. Usually, these are created by their complex customer requirements, complex multi-location and cloud architectures, virtualized infrastructure and their need for simultaneous deployment of multiple new applications. All this creates an expanded attack surface that allows constantly evolving and innovative cyber-threats to find their way in. Some of these attacks can be severe enough to cause expenditures up to $11 million with a single breach.

The healthcare industry today relies primarily on technology. It requires technology not only for providing increasingly sophisticated healthcare related services, but also for communicating with various departments and facilities within the organization. With the implementation of communication and information technology, the healthcare industry has introduced new levels of efficiency. That in turn, has led to noticeable cost-saving measures across the board. Therefore, it is very important to maintain properly the network that delivers the information employees need when they need it without any glitches.

When selecting a vendor for a specific need, healthcare providers do not make the decision in a vacuum. Before introducing a new product, they need to consider the potential domino effect that may affect other technologies and applications. Therefore, when Catholic Health Systems needed a new networking product, they clarified that they had specific requirements, pertaining to both environment and budget, and that they knew there would be a repercussion on other areas of IT within the organization.

THE REQUIREMENT

Catholic Health is a non-profit healthcare system that includes 8,600 employees and 1,000 acute care beds. They cater to rehab and lab services across 14 cities, providing long-term care, primary care and acute care. It was imperative that they implement a robust, secure network. For making its decision, the organization wanted to bring security and access to its medical imaging systems and its EMR or electronic medical records. According to a press release, Catholic Health made a decision to pick up MetaFabric, a Juniper Networks product, to allow it to meet HIPAA compliance regulations. The security lessons learned may be useful for other organizations, especially since Catholic Health made their decision on a fairly tight budget.

Although several next-generation technologies exist in the market for organizations that have defined needs and flush with large budgets, it is a fact that not all healthcare organizations are deploying these new-age products. Therefore, organizations such as Catholic Health, with multiple on-premise data centers, must focus on the best network switches for simplifying their IT department's day-to-day work.

The data centers of Catholic Health employ both virtual and physical environments within them, which makes it necessary for the data center to stay agile. Another important requirement is having adjacent security technologies together with solid networking infrastructure. Catholic found their requirements were completely met with the network firewall technologies, again from Juniper. As part of the implementation, Catholic also bought prevention appliances, intrusion detection and remote access from Juniper.

According to Catholic Health, their mission is to provide their patients with a positive experience of patient care. They feel technology to be a huge enabler of better care, since it provides the staff with an easily adaptable and agile network. That allows the patients to receive effective and pinpointed healthcare.

Selecting a vendor is never about a single item. Networking products have complicated inter-connectivity between technologies, which makes the selection an increasingly challenging process. While organizations need to account for devices connected or connecting to their network, they also need to control what is being fed into the network. On the other hand, the information flowing out from their network may be a separate story altogether. Catholic Health decided to pick Juniper's products as it specifically met their precise set of needs. However, other organizations may have different requirements and different vendor prerequisites, so the same products may not be as good of a fit.

THE SOLUTION

Juniper Network's MetaFabric architecture provides the deployment and delivery of applications for clouds and multiple sites. It provides a combination of powerful platforms for routing, switching and security, using integration with the technology ecosystem, leveraging network orchestration, programmable systems, feature-rich silicon, open APIs and SDN. This allows Catholic Health to simplify and scale its data center operations to support the life critical applications throughout the organization.

Juniper's products have provided the data centers of Catholic Health with advanced security capabilities, exceeding those available with traditional methods. Typically, traditional methods respond to, detect and prevent targeted threats adaptively. Juniper uses an innovative technology of intrusion deception that detects the attacker early in it reconnaissance phase. It then proceeds to respond by fingerprinting the offending device, rendering it useless in further attacks.

Juniper has switching networks suitable for high performance data centers. Apart from providing advanced security capabilities, these networks are not hampered by Firefly Perimeter, SRX Series Services Gateways or the Firefly Host. For automating creation and enforcement of policy, there is the Junos Space Security Director, which also helps improve the reach, accuracy and ease of the administration of security policy at the user, application and server levels.

THE BENEFITS

Juniper's solutions have securely delivered greater levels of business agility and performance to Catholic Health. The wide-ranging, preventative security tools, in conjunction with high-performing and scalable data center solutions, have helped change the economic model of modern cyber-attacks.

The MetaFabric architecture provides three pillars to solve the complexity of creating an efficient network in the multifactorial data center landscape of Catholic Health. These include:

Simplicity: Enabling ease of deployment, operations and management of the network, without causing service interruptions

Openness: Maximizing flexibility by eliminating vendor lock-in and integrating with any data center environment

Efficiency: Saving time and improving the performance of the network through actionable insights and data analytics.

The solution also delivers the latest operations and network architecture requirements including hybrid, public and private cloud computing, server virtualization and SDN transformation projects. Most importantly, it provides a security platform capable of addressing threats by adapting to responding, detecting and defending to targeted threats.

ELECTRONIC HEALTH RECORDS—THEIR PRIVACY AND SECURITY

Fast-changing trends in healthcare and tools used therein are providing improved coordination and better care for everyone. Most doctors now enter notes on a laptop or a computer, these devices are logged into an EHR or electronic health record. EHRs enable healthcare providers to offer improved and coordinated care, while simultaneously providing them access to the health information of their patients. This makes it easier for everyone to remain better informed thus providing the right kind of healthcare to the patient.

However, the use of EHRs does raise several questions and concerns. Patients understandably have concerns regarding the privacy and security of their health information. Who is accessing the information on my EHR? How can I examine the information on my record and ensure that it is accurate? Is it protected from hacking, theft and loss? Will I be informed and if so, what should I do if my information has become compromised?

OCR or the Office for Civil Rights, under HHS, enforces the HIPAA Privacy and Security Rules. Entities covered under HIPAA must comply with these rules and be accountable for the security and privacy of the health information of their patients. EHRs allow healthcare providers to improve the quality and efficiency of their care by using information more effectively. However, EHRs do not change the obligation that healthcare providers have for keeping protected health information of their patients private and secure.

PATIENT RIGHTS

Most patients understand some health privacy jargon such as the "Notice of Privacy Practice" or "HIPAA". However, they often have little knowledge about their rights under the HIPAA Privacy and Security Rules and more importantly, the relationship these rules have with EHRs.

According to the HIPAA Privacy Rule, a patient has rights over his or her own health information, regardless of the form it is stored in. So, irrespective of whether the record is in electronic form, paper or any other, under the Privacy Rule, a patient has the right:

- To get and to see a copy of his or her own medical record

- To request and have any mistakes corrected

- To receive a notice about how his or her health information is to be used and shared

- To declare how and where he or she wants the healthcare provider to contact them

- To file a complaint if he or she notices a violation of these rights

The doctor's office or the hospital will give the patient these rights spelled out in the Notice of Privacy Practices. The patient may also receive this notice as a part of the health plan sent to them in the mail.

SAFEGUARDS REQUIRED FROM THE HEALTHCARE PROVIDERS

According to the HIPAA Security Rule, healthcare providers are required to set up physical, administrative, and technical safeguards for protecting the electronic health information of their patients. This is specific to EHRs and relates to protecting the data stored in them. EHR systems may also have some safety measures built into them, including:

- Limiting the access to patient information through "Access controls" such as passwords and PIN numbers

- Keeping the stored information encrypted. "Encrypting" means the health information cannot be read or understood by anyone other than by the person who can 'decrypt' it, using a special "key" given only to authorized individuals.

- Maintaining an "audit trail" by recording who accessed what information and what changes were made and when

In certain circumstances, if a patient's data is seen by someone who is not authorized, federal law mandates that doctors, hospitals and other healthcare providers notify the patient of the "breach" of their health information. This mandate helps to keep the healthcare providers accountable and lets patients know if anything has gone wrong with the protection of their data.

OCR's objective is to ensure that healthcare professionals maintain the privacy and security of their patient's health information. OCR assures patients about their rights, helps in understanding them, the actions to be taken if these rights are violated, and the way health information may be protected under the law.

WHAT YOU NEED TO KNOW ABOUT VIEWING, DOWNLOADING AND TRANSMITTING—2014 REQUIREMENTS

There is colossal confusion about what to expect when viewing, downloading, and transmitting patient data as part of the Meaningful Use requirements.

According to the HITECH Act, healthcare entities must adopt implementation of electronic health records through Meaningful Use. There are three stages of the program and Meaningful Use means providers must demonstrate the use of certified EHR technology so that they achieve significant measurements in quality and quantity.

MEANINGFUL USE STAGE 1

Stage 1 began in 2011, and set the basic functionality for EHRs. The focus is primarily on healthcare providers who capture patient data and share it either with the patient or with other healthcare professionals. Eligible hospitals, professionals and critical access hospitals must successfully attest to two reporting periods of stage 1, before they can move to stage 2.

MEANINGFUL USE STAGE 2

Stage 2 begins in 2014, and uses advanced clinical processes. The focus is primarily on health information exchange between providers. It promotes patient engagement by giving them secure online access to their health information.

MEANINGFUL USE STAGE 3

Stage 3 is set to begin in 2016, but the rule is not yet finalized.

MEANINGFUL USE AND IMPLEMENTATION

Implementation of patient engagement functionality in EHRs throws up challenges and opportunities because of new requirements, such as Meaningful Use, when a certain percentage of patients VDT or view, download and transmit their health information.

All hospitals and providers that have complied with Meaningful Use in 2014 must implement the VDT capabilities for their patients. However, there is still quite a bit of confusion regarding what to expect for VDT. Those still in Stage 1 must attest for access, while those in Stage 2 must attest for use. In the VDT measure definition, use of the term "online access" refers to all the three capabilities—view, download and transmit.

ATTESTING FOR ACCESS

The healthcare organization must provide the ability for fifty percent of their patients to view their data, download it in both machine and human readable formats and transmit their data electronically.

None of these three functions is optional, and patients must have access to all the three functions as long as the provider's reporting period remains valid.

The CMS and ONC rules explicitly define the types of data that patients can view, how quickly they can view it after an encounter with an institution or a provider, and the format that the data must be available in for downloading and transmitting. For example, for downloading and transmitting, the defined machine-readable format is the Consolidated CDA.

ATTESTING FOR USE

Within the specified reporting period, five percent of all patients must be able to view, download and or transmit their healthcare information. Although any combination of VDT may be used, institutions or providers do not have the option to turn off the other functions.

USE OF DIRECT PROTOCOL

Another confusion pertains to whether the transmit portion of VDT requires Direct Protocol. As part of the ONC certification, Direct is mandatory for patient transmit; therefore, every certified EHR has this functionality built-in. However, for CMS attestation, providers are free to use an alternate form of transmit in order to achieve the 50 percent "access" and five percent "use" requirements.

Since Direct is built-in into all certified EHRs, the Direct Protocol is at this point the simplest way to meet the transmit requirements. Direct is also the same transmitting method adopted by providers to comply with requirements of Transition of Care. Additionally, several patient-facing applications and tools are currently implementing this as well.

As patients using VDT are free to choose where they will transmit their own health information, the transmit method, including

Direct Protocol, must be implemented in a way that a patient can designate any Direct address, consumer application or tool that will receive their data.

CONCLUSION

2014 will be a significant year not only for Meaningful Use, but also for the community of patients, caregivers, providers and entrepreneurs looking for innovative ways to create tools to facilitate patient access to their own health information.

HUMAN ERROR & ๒.
DATA SECURITY THRE๒.

The greatest threat of a healthcare data breach is from employee negligence.

The fourth annual Patient Privacy and Data Security Study conducted by the Ponemon Institute substantiated some facts about healthcare data breach that were already known. The study reviewed some new and expanded threats relating to patient data security and privacy. Of the 91 healthcare organizations who participated in this study, they concluded that more than 75 percent of the organizations view negligence from employees as the greatest threat to data breach, and that human error remains the biggest source of breaches for healthcare data.

SIGNIFICANT FINDINGS OF THE REPORT

Ponemon conducted their research by interviewing 388 healthcare providers. A total of 91 healthcare organizations were involved and, which is 11 more than their sample size in 2012. Some topics covered in the study include:

- The need to reduce internal as well as external threats
- HIPAA compliance trends
- Cloud security
- Mobile device security

ing negligence, 41 percent of the participating organizations their biggest security concerns were the use of public cloud ices, 40 percent listed mobile device insecurity and 39 percent re insecure over cyber-attacks.

An astounding figure of 90 percent of the respondents in the study confirmed they have had at least one data breach within the last two years. Of that 90 percent, 38 percent confirmed having more than five data breaches over the same two-year period; last year this figure was 45 percent. According to the study, the only positive result favorable to the healthcare industry is that data breach cost and frequency has declined slightly over the past one year as compared to the previous years. The chairman and founder of the Ponemon Institute, Larry Ponemon, concluded that this was an indication that organizations are making modest but good progress in managing sensitive patient data.

The primary causes of breaches were as follows:

- Computing devices, lost or stolen—49 percent

- Unintentional actions or mistakes by employees—46 percent

- Snafus from third-parties—41 percent

Assessing it in economic terms, the study reported that data breaches had cost the healthcare organizations between less than $10,000 to more than $1 million. As calculated by Ponemon, the average monetary impact of data breaches is in the $2 million range over a two year period, for the healthcare organizations represented in the study. Compared to last year, this is actually down from 2.4 million. The figure is down partly because of the decrease in the size of the breaches, since the average number of stolen or lost records per breach came down to 2,150; it was 3,000 records earlier. Ponemon estimates $188 per record, which makes the cost of one breach $404,200.

Of the critical themes mentioned in the report, three of them were HIPAA compliance, cloud security and mobile security. The report claims that nearly 88 percent of the healthcare organizations allow their medical staff and employees to bring and use their own devices (BYOD). However, over half of the organizations are not confident of the security of these personally owned mobile devices.

Furthermore, only 23 percent of the organizations confirmed that they insist on anti-malware/anti-virus software being resident on the mobile device before it is connected to their network. Only 22 percent require that mobile devices be scanned for viruses and malware before connection, and only 14 percent want removal of all mobile applications that present a security threat. Healthcare organizations have started to realize that with more tablets and smartphones now being used in the workplace, one of the greatest sources of data breach is the loss of devices.

The use of cloud for backup and storage, file sharing applications, document sharing and collaboration and business applications has increased to 40 percent; the figure was 32 percent last year. However, only one third expressed having any real confidence over the security of information stored in a public cloud environment.

While only 49 percent of the respondents said they are either not compliant or only partially compliant with HIPAA, 51 percent confirmed they are fully compliant with HIPAA requirements. Moreover, 39 percent said that their incident assessment process is non-effective primarily due to lack of consistency and their inability to scale their processes.

Only 33 percent were somewhat confident and 40 percent were not confident at all that their business associates had the capability to detect, perform an incident risk assessment and notify the organization in the event of an information breach incident, as required under the BAA or business associate agreement. While 44 percent of the healthcare organizations say the HIPAA Omnibus Rule has affected their programs, 41 percent claim no change and 15 percent are yet undecided.

Some entities covered by HIPAA and HITECH are adopting a strategy of trying to be just compliant without caring for the broader, cross-industry security risks. However, organizations are learning that compliance with HIPAA does not necessarily translate into good security for the organization.

Organizations are striving to achieve the requirements of HHS or OCR, whether it is through better procedures, policies or training. However, they are missing the boat because healthcare ecosystems are increasingly becoming more complex and this is evident in several recent incidents. It is not enough to rely on telling an employee that they are responsible for PHI protection, necessary technologies and tools must be in place. For example, encryption makes it less likely for an employee to do anything to protect the data.

SOME OTHER KEY FINDINGS

Of the healthcare organizations represented in the report, 69 percent believe that ACA increases the risk to patient privacy and security significantly. Primary concerns were, 75 percent worried about insecure exchange of patient information between healthcare providers and government, 65 percent cite the risk to be patient data on insecure databases and 63 percent on patient registration on insecure websites.

While 51 percent of the organizations are part of an ACO or Accountable Care Organization, 66 percent say the risk to patient security and privacy has increased because of an increase in the exchange of patient health information among participants.

Only 32 percent of the respondents are confident about the security and privacy of patient data being shared on HIEs, while 40 percent are not confident at all.

Only 25 percent of the respondents or less than half of the organizations in the study confirmed they are fully compliant with the AOD or Accounting of Disclosure requirement; 23 percent are nearly in full compliance.

Almost all respondents deemed that medical files, insurance records and billing records are the ones most likely to be lost or stolen.

OVERCOMING CHALLENGES FACED DURING HEALTH INFORMATION EXCHANGES

State Privacy Rules and Patient Record Matching are highlighted as the most serious hurdles faced during Health Information Exchanges.

The Government Accountability Office, in their latest report, has pointed to the toughest ongoing challenges facing the health information exchange. The major hurdles among them being complying with privacy rules that differ from state to state, and matching patients to all the appropriate electronic records.

Ongoing HIE efforts in four states resulted in the GAO report, which is based on interviews with healthcare providers and other stakeholders. Key challenges faced by those interviewed included issues related to difficulties in matching patients to their records, concerns about privacy rules varying among states, insufficient standards and costs associated with health information exchange. GAO interviewed healthcare providers and other stakeholders in Massachusetts, Minnesota, North Carolina and Georgia, in the summer months of 2013.

Some aspects of these key challenges are being addressed by several ongoing initiatives including programs by two units of the DHHS or the Department of Health and Human Services. These are the Office of the National Coordinator for Health Information Technology and the Centers for Medicare and Medicaid Services. However, concerns in these areas persist. Several providers substantiate this. They informed GAO about their difficulty in exchanging specific types of health information because the health data standards are not sufficient.

DIFFICULTY IN EXCHANGING ACROSS STATE LINES

Some providers have reported facing difficulty when exchanging data with entities in other states because privacy rules vary across states; the absence of clarity in the rules increases the difficulty.

Patients living on the state borders, such as in the Tri-state area of Connecticut, New Jersey and New York, are the ones for whom the complexness of differing state privacy rules create the major hurdles most frequently.

While it is understood that these challenges do make data exchange difficult across regions, HHS still targets a nationwide health information exchange, since the HITECH Act calls for it. According to the new head of ONC, Karen DeSalvo, it is possible to attain health information exchange on a national level within the next three years. However, matching patients to all their proper records is critical for data security, patient safety and privacy concerns and must be addressed beforehand.

DIFFICULTIES WITH PATIENT DATA MATCHING

Patient matching is a technological challenge for health information exchange. It is necessary to make sure the data flows smartly, by sorting out the origin of the information and its ultimate destination. Patient matching is specifically important as doctors proceed to integrate data.

The actual issue lies in making sure that all the correct data coming from multiple sources relate to the right patient and that it reaches the correct clinician at the appropriate time. The process involves safety as much as it does security.

ONC has launched a patient ID collaborative initiative for addressing the issue of matching patients to all the right records. The goal is to improve patient matching based on current approaches used by selected stakeholders. They intend to identify algorithms and key attributes for matching patients to their records. ONC will define the best practices or processes in support of the identified key attributes.

According to GAO, ONC completed the first phase of their initiative by releasing a report that contained recommendations for patient matching. This report was slated for a possible inclusion in the electronic health record incentive program at Stage 3 of the HITECH Act, together with the 2015 edition of the standards and certification criteria.

According to the ONC report, a strategy document developed and issued by HHS in August 2013, describes its expectations for advancing electronic health information exchange. The strategy document identifies the principles required for guiding future actions in addressing the key challenges that the healthcare providers and stakeholders have identified. However, the HHS strategy does not specifically mention any such action, the prioritization of the actions, any milestones that need to be achieved or the period when such milestones need to be accomplished.

Consequently, the report only points out that ONC and CMS must develop and prioritize specific actions for advancing health information exchange. It also calls for the agencies to set up milestones with periods for the actions, so that the progress towards advancing exchange may be gauged in a more thorough manner, and appropriate adjustments made over time.

WHAT ARE THE SIGNS OF PROGRESS?

Although security and privacy matters are among the topmost concerns for health information exchange, progress is slowly by surely being made in those areas. For example, legal teams are improving their trust agreements. The teams represent health information exchange organizations, physician practices, hospitals and care organizations that are accountable. The agreements spell out the terms for sharing patient information among the entities. That is how they are holding up the basis of HIE—trust and stewardship of data.

Technology vendors are tackling the patient matching issue. On the Internet, identity matching is a common e-commerce practice. Although for HIE it is still an issue, identity management solutions are out there, and vendors need to leverage that. Experts feel that although patient matching may never reach absolute perfection, it is likely to get better with the growing demand for HIE.

However, the lack of industry wide interoperability standards is a more challenging hurdle for HIE. Most healthcare organizations find that setting up the HIE may not be cost-prohibitive. However, getting everyone to connect is a bigger headache. For example, a vendor solution for setting up an HIE may cost an organization $1 million, but that does not guarantee the healthcare organization will be able to interface its systems with an exchange without spending thousands more, especially due to the lack of interoperability standards.

In stage 3 of the electronic health records incentive program of the HITECH Act, HHS is working on integration of electronic directories of providers and patients and on standards for point-to-point data queries. The government wants to add value in these two areas. It has created the health information exchange workgroup and the privacy and security tiger team as two HIT Policy Committee advisory panels.

The EHR incentive program has done a commendable job of giving providers the necessary tools that has kick-started the demand for interoperability and now, the market must take it forward. The government is assisting by funding the startup and early operations of many HIEs, including those of statewide efforts launched under the HITECH Act. However, the funding may not continue forever, and HIEs must devise a plan for financial sustainability, possibly by charging the participating healthcare organizations a subscribing fee.

PHI DATA BREACH THROUGH MISSING FLASH DRIVES IN MEDICAL CENTERS

Technical equipment with internal memory should be handled carefully as it can retain information such as PHI.

DATA BREACH AT THE ORLANDO HEALTH'S ARNOLD PALMER MEDICAL CENTER

According to the Orlando Health's Arnold Palmer Medical Center Sentinel report, a flash drive containing patients' data was lost in Jan 2014. While the drive did not include patients' financial data or their Social Security numbers on it, it did however include names, dates of birth, assigned medical record numbers, birth weights, gestational ages, and dates of hospitalizations. The medical center does not suspect the device was stolen, but only lost.

A flash drive is a small memory device for storing information and is used on a computer. The device misplaced at Arnold Palmer contained limited data of 586 children treated there between 2009 and 2013. The medical center is treating the lost device as a data security breach. Although there is no evidence of any information on the flash drive being accessed or any unauthorized individual using it, as a precautionary measure, Orlando Health has notified affected families.

According to the hospital, upon learning of the incident, the staff immediately conducted a search to locate the flash drive, but was unsuccessful in their attempt. One speculation was that the employee may have placed the thumb drive in the pocket of his/her lab coat. When the lab coat was discarded, the drive may have also mistakenly been thrown away as well. To prevent similar incidents from happening again, the hospital is reeducating its employees regarding the importance of handling patient information securely and the use of portable memory devices.

THE KAISER PERMANENTE PRIVACY BREACH AT ANAHEIM MEDICAL CENTER

A privacy breach at the Anaheim Medical Center in California has exposed the personal information of nearly 50,000 patients. Healthcare provider Kaiser Permanente filed a data breach notification letter with the California Attorney General's office, informing them that the personal information was in a USB flash drive that went missing.

The misplaced flash drive contained names, medical record numbers, dates of birth and medications of patients who had obtained health care at the Anaheim facility of the company. Anaheim Medical Center discovered the loss and reported it to Kaiser Permanente on Sept 25th. The company sent out letters to affected patients a month after the actual event.

THE STRUGGLE TO MAINTAIN COMPLIANCE

Such breaches are one in several healthcare related data losses. Solution providers say these incidents are increasing in frequency because of the growing complexity of the systems most providers are using. Hospitals usually have a myriad of partners involved in delivering healthcare, which makes it difficult for these clinics and medical offices to maintain compliance with healthcare regulations. According to 4A Security, a systems integrator and information security risk and compliance consultancy based in New York, maintaining compliance with HIPAA is a difficult task when data has to be controlled in association with partners and other contractors.

Information at any place is growing exponentially, but the compliance burden remains the same whether it is a small medical unit or a hospital with several locations in different areas of the country. Compounding this matter is that lack of clear cut administrative policy enforcement tool.

Healthcare organizations must be careful when handling any technical equipment designed to retain information. HIPAA covered entities are responsible for ensuring protection for all personal information of their patients.

CONSEQUENCES OF FAILURE TO COMPLY

Since 2013, HIPAA has significantly increased the fines associated with failure to comply. This came about following the movement of enforcement to the OCR under the Department of Health and Human Services. Another update to HIPAA came under the Omnibus Rule which then increased the penalties even further, extending it to all business associates of healthcare providers. Under the Omnibus Rule, violations are categorized in a tier-based system and fines can run from $1,000 to $1.5 million, per violation.

REMEDIATING THE RISK AND ADDRESSING SECURITY ISSUES

Remediating risk within a healthcare organization and addressing security issues within the medical environment takes time and constant vigilance. The security programs in most healthcare organizations are still in their infancy, and the industry is facing complex issues as organizations race to digitize medical records. According to MMIC, the largest medical liability insurer in the Midwest owned by policyholders, medical institutions are overwhelmed about how best to implement safeguards while simultaneously addressing compliance.

Although stolen smartphones and laptops are typically associated with criminals interested in reselling the physical device, cybercriminals are increasingly targeting healthcare organizations in order to steal sensitive data.

MARKET VALUE OF HEALTH INSURANCE DATA

Dell SecureWorks, in a recent study has uncovered an underground market for health insurance data valued at millions of dollars. Criminals use brokered online forums and chat rooms for buying and selling patient information including Social Security numbers, health insurance credentials and others. The researchers found that the data is used to help illegal foreigners, criminals and immigrants in order to obtain specialized medical care in the US.

PRACTICAL TIPS FOR HANDLING TECHNICAL EQUIPMENT CONTAINING INTERNAL MEMORY

Technical machines and equipment used today typically contain hard drives and internal memory chips that can store data. In several cases, the stored data may be difficult to erase. Examples of such equipment are computers, servers, fax machines, scanners and photocopiers. Additionally, there may also be communication monitoring systems and security videos maintaining such information on backup tapes and modern cellphones.

Typically, such instruments and devices are traded in for newer models. However, in order to prevent leakage of information, it is necessary to completely clean or destroy all data contained within that machine, using professional help if necessary, before they are traded in for a newer model, sold or even discarded.

The following steps are helpful when handling protected health information in an organization:

- Make sure that encryption is used on all types of electronic media by which patient health information is transferred. This may include flash or thumb drives, DVDs, CD ROMs, backup tapes and several types of mini hard drives.

- Preferably, patient information should remain at the work site. If it is necessary to work on the data from a remote location, a secure and encrypted Internet connection must be used for accessing the work database. Saving the data or work on a laptop hard drives or other removable media must be avoided.

- Never leave any media or laptop in a car that will be worked on by a mechanic, car wash or while entering a store. Thieves are aware of such locations and wait for careless individuals to slip up.

OPTIONS FOR ENCRYPTION OF PERSONAL HEALTH INFORMATION

Changes made to the HIPAA Security Rule raise questions about encryption among physicians and other healthcare professionals.

As part of the American Recovery and Reinvestment act of 2009, the HITECH Act or the Health Information Technology for Economic and Clinical Health Act has made several changes to the HIPAA Security Rule. These changes, related to encryption, have raised several questions among physicians and other professionals in the healthcare industry along with other HIPAA-covered entities and their business associates. It should also be noted that many states have laws and regulations that are more demanding than the federal requirements outlined here and that physicians must confirm if any local requirements apply.

ARE CHANGES TO THE HIPAA SECURITY RULE APPLICABLE TO SMALL PRACTICES?

According to the change in the HIPAA Security Rule, it is necessary for HIPAA-covered entities and their business associates to provide notification in case they face a breach of unsecured PHI or protected health information. For example, if a hacker were to gain access to the computer system, tablet, laptop, PDA, etc, belonging to a physician's practice and it contained PHI that was not encrypted; the practice would then have to notify both the patients and the Department of HHS or Health and Human Services of the breach. Some states require the physician's practice to notify the media as well. Therefore, lack of compliance may result not only in reputational harm to the practice; it might also risk exposure of the most sensitive nature belonging to patients within that practice.

HOW TO MITIGATE THE BREACH NOTIFICATION REQUIREMENTS OF HIPAA?

Physicians can secure their data through encryption to avoid these notification requirements. If they have stored and transmitted the electronic PHI or ePHI in encrypted form, then they need not notify the patients, even in case of a security breach. Physicians and other HIPAA-covered entities including their business associates can follow the standards established by NIST or National Institute of Standards and Technology. The standards describe the technology and methods to be used for rendering ePHI unreadable, unusable or indecipherable to individuals unauthorized to access them.

The extremely technical guidance, Special Publication 800-66-Revision 1, recommends that physicians and software vendors work together to make sure that the electronic devices and computers used have acceptable software loaded for encryption. The HIPAA Omnibus Rule confirms that if the encryption and destruction of data were consistent with NIST guidelines, there would be no need for notification in the event of a breach. While covered entities and business associates do not need to follow this guidance, if the physician's practice implements the specified technologies and methods, it can avoid having to comply with the breach notification requirements of HIPAA.

WHAT EXACTLY IS ENCRYPTION?

In layman's terms, encryption is the process of storing the patient data behind a locked door, access to which is only possible with a suitable key. Encryption transforms information to make it unreadable to those who do not have the key. That means even if a hacker were to gain access to a computer containing PHI, he or she will be unable to read or interpret that information and the patient's privacy will remain protected.

HOW IS DATA ENCRYPTED?

Vendors use special computer programs or specially designed computer hardware for implementing encryption of data. By applying a mathematical algorithm, these programs or devices convert the PHI in the computer to a scrambled form of the original data. This can be restored to its original form with the help of a key, which the legitimate user possesses and uses when he needs to access the data. The key causes a reversing of the scrambling process and the scrambling program or device restores the data to its original form. Those who possess the key can only initiate the unscrambling process.

WHAT ARE THE DIFFERENT ALGORITHMS USED FOR ENCRYPTION?

Various inventors have developed different types of special mathematical algorithms for encryption. These algorithms are like recipes in that they specify the ingredients and the specific steps needed to be taken to produce the encrypted data; the ingredients are the key and the plaintext data. Among the many types of algorithms available, most notable are: Serpent, MARS, Twofish, Rijndael, Triple-DES and DES.

WHAT IS THE DIFFERENCE BETWEEN SECRET, PUBLIC AND PRIVATE KEYS?

Encryption algorithms use many types of keys. Traditional encryption schemes used the same secret key to both encrypt and decrypt data. Newer methods of encryption, also known as public-key algorithms, use a public key for encrypting information, and only its corresponding private key can decrypt it. Think of this as a post office box. Anyone can drop letters in the box, but only the owner can open the box to take them out.

DOES ENCRYPTION WORK ONLY ON SPECIAL TYPES OF DATA?

Any type of data, whether it is at rest or in transit, can be encrypted. That means you can encrypt files on computer storage devices, since they are at rest, and data being transferred via the Internet, since they are in transit. Any type of plaintext files, spreadsheets, PDF documents, images and any other kind of information in the computer can be encrypted, including databases and information stored on back-up media.

WHAT DATA FROM A PHYSICIAN PRACTICE SHOULD BE ENCRYPTED?

Any individual file containing PHI and stored electronically, also called ePHI, should be encrypted. Data that a physician practice requires to encrypt includes the practice management system, claims payment appeals, electronic medical records, scanned images, copies of remittance advices, emails that contain ePHI, transmitted ePHI, such as claims sent to the clearinghouse, and any back-ups that are made of the electronic system and or files.

IS IT NECESSARY TO ENCRYPT EMAILS CONTAINING EPHI?

Although legally, physicians can send PHI through non-secure emails, this is not recommended, since an unauthorized party can breach the information. Therefore, recommendations from the AMA are that physicians should use encrypted email for sending PHI. Unlike a sealed letter or a packet, emails are rather like a post-card. Although people are not supposed to read a postcard while it is in transit, one can never be sure if someone has not already read it.

Several tools are available to encrypt emails before sending them. However, if a physician prefers using unsecure emails for communication, they should seek written permission from the patient for doing so while explaining the risks involved.

IS IT NECESSARY TO ENCRYPT EPHI ACCESSED VIA THE INTERNET?

It is necessary to encrypt ePHI accessed via the Internet. Content published on the Internet is available to the public to read. PHI is not public information, and it is not meant for all to read. Therefore, it needs to be encrypted before it goes on the Internet. Encrypted PHI is made available on a website with a technology known as SSL/TLS or as secure sockets layer/transport layer security.

HOW DIFFICULT IS IT TO ENCRYPT DATA?

The method chosen for encryption of sensitive data determines the difficulty of the process. Typically, the system administrator takes up the initial investment of time and effort needed to install and configure the product. For physician practices that do not make use of system administrators may need to work with the contractor for setting up the encryption product initially.

Once implemented, the process of encryption and decryption of data should be almost automatic. Minimal user involvement is required, mainly for specifying which data items need to be encrypted. Provided the installation and set-up have been completed properly, the encryption and decryption process should not impact normal operations or workflow in any way.

HOW DOES ONE ENCRYPT THE DATA ON THEIR COMPUTER?

There are different products to choose from. EFS or Encrypting File System from Microsoft simply changes the properties of the folder containing the sensitive data. The Microsoft Windows operating system also has an additional security feature known as the BitLocker Drive Encryption. Those using Mac OS X can use File Vault 2, which is similar in functionality to BitLocker. Linux users have a vast choice among several types of file and full disk encryption options freely available.

IS ENCRYPTION EXPENSIVE?

Depending on whether one is using a free or a non-free product, the expenses of encryption will vary from zero to quite expensive depending on its sophistication level. Most major operating system vendors already include cryptographic utility programs with their software. Other programs may be downloaded and installed freely such as TrueCrypt. All web servers and browsers already use SSL/TLS technology that satisfies the needs of ePHI encryption.

On the other hand, HSMs or hardware security modules are very expensive devices. The choice depends on several factors such as the encryption speed, strength, available technical support and ease of use.

WHAT DOES NIST RECOMMEND?

NIST specifies a preference for ECC or elliptic curve cryptography as it is stronger and faster than most known public key algorithms such as RSA and AES.

WHERE IS THE BEST PLACE FOR KEEPING THE KEYS?

A number of different places are specified for safekeeping the keys used for encryption and decryption of PHI. These places include USB flash drives, smart cards and CDs. Sometimes, a computer network may have a key-server device for storing keys. Some keys do not require storing at all, instead it is regenerated as a one-time number when needed.

Keeping keys on the same computer that contains the encrypted data is considered extremely unsafe, and HHS does not allow an exemption from the requirements of breach notification if keys were on the same device as the encrypted data.

Encryption products typically allow a choice of where the keys should be kept as an option while installing or configuring. It is important to know where the keys are kept.

WHAT IF A HACKER FINDS THE KEY?

The encrypted data is no longer safe if the key falls into the hands of a hacker.

DOES THE SIZE OF THE KEY MAKE A DIFFERENCE?

Key size is an indication of how strong the encryption is. Generally, the longer the key size, the better is the protection. For example, a 256-bit key has better protection features than a 128-bit key. However, a longer key can make the performance slower. Therefore, the trade-off is between performance and security.

WHAT CAN GO WRONG?

A potential problem is losing the encryption key and being unable to retrieve the encrypted data when needed. Therefore, it would be wise to ensure there is a backup copy of all encryption keys in a safe place.

Do not use old encryption algorithms since they may have been compromised and encrypted data will not be safe using them.

FIPS ENCRYPTION AND HIPAA REQUIREMENTS

The US Department of Defense mandates FIPS for encryption as a powerful security solution to reduce risks and cost.

To comply with the HIPAA standard, healthcare providers and their business associates are increasingly turning to verified and certified network security products offered by leaders in networking such as Cisco. Encryption products recommended by the HHS or the US Department of Health and Human Services include those certified by the FIPS or Federal Information Process Standard for protecting healthcare data. FIPS 140-2 is already mandated by DoD or the US Department of Defense, and it is a powerful security solution for reducing risks as well as costs.

This is the perfect time to consider an investment in information security, as HITECH is currently offering economic stimulus funding to help providers achieve meaningful use of their medical information.

THE RISKS OF NONCOMPLIANCE

According to the National Preparedness Report, released by FEMA or the Federal Emergency Management Agency, the healthcare industry is well set to face several types of emergencies and problems. However, the same report also mentions that most healthcare providers and their business associates are not ready to handle any type of cyber security attack. Only about 40% of state officials were of the view that they were adequately prepared.

According to the same report, almost 66% of all US companies sustained cyber-attacks over the past six years, with the number of reported attacks in the US going up by 650%. This tumultuous environment makes compliance with HIPAA requirements a top priority. Prior to 2009, a general consensus in the healthcare industry was that HIPAA was not rigorously enforced. With the enactment of HITECH, healthcare providers can now be penalized for willful neglect unless they provide evidence of compliance to the Act. These penalties may go up to $250,000, and fines for uncorrected violations may reach $1.5 million.

HHS will now conduct periodic audits of covered entities and their business associates. That means all healthcare providers must have suitable systems in place for monitoring business practices and relationships so that consistent security for all medical information is assured.

TYPES OF CYBER SECURITY RISKS FACED BY THE HEALTHCARE INDUSTRY

The healthcare industry may face various types of threats, for instance:

- A virus attack crippled all computer systems in the Kern Medical Center in Bakersfield, CA. It took the hospital nearly 10 days to get all doctors and nurses back online.

- At a Chicago hospital, computers, attacked by a malware, were forced into a botnet under the control of a hacker. A year later, they are still struggling with the consequences of the attack.

- A computer tape containing unencrypted PHI or personal health information was stolen from the car of an employee of DoD, which is now facing a multi-billion dollar lawsuit because of the theft.

- Pharmacy dispensing cabinets, glucometers and PACS or picture archiving and communication systems, belonging to the Veterans Administrations, were hacked along with other medical devices and wireless networks. They waged a two-year war against the intrusions.

ADVANTAGES OF COMPLIANCE

When medical information is managed securely, it protects patients against discrimination and identity theft, including risks of life-threatening interference with medical devices or equipment. Simultaneously, data needs to be available quickly as needed, for example, to emergency personnel. If the business is to remain competitive, the following benefits are critical:

- Patients should get better quality of care
- Outcome of patients should improve
- Workflow efficiency and productivity must increase
- Better information should be available at the point of care
- Doctors and nurses should have improved and integrated communication methods.

ENCRYPTION IS THE KEY TO COMPLIANCE

For mitigating these risks, healthcare service providers must assure that information across their network is inaccessible to unauthorized users. HHS has issued guidelines recommending the use of encryption technologies compliant with the FIPS 140-2 standard. Cisco is offering its NGE or next generation encryption, which is fully compliant with FIPS-140, and claims that the security level provided by NGE will remain fully compliant even after 2030.

Encryption is the process of converting the message in a file or document into an unreadable format before it can be sent, and decrypting it at the other end to return it to a readable state. For meeting the requirements of the HITECH Act, the main service provider must implement encryption within both its network and the networks of its associated partners.

Success of the encryption process depends on the strength of its algorithm and the security of the decryption key, when data is either in motion or at rest. Instances of data in motion are when it is moving through a network or via wireless transmission. Instances of data at rest are when data is residing in file systems, databases or in other structured methods of storage.

Almost all healthcare organizations have Internet access, and that makes it mandatory for them to implement encryption methods. Electronic transactions in healthcare are increasing, including electronic communications and e-prescribing. Additionally, most medical organizations now use open systems and they do need to implement encryption tools.

HOW DOES FIPS 140-2 HELP SECURE INFORMATION?

The US and Canadian governments have defined FIPS 140-2 as a standard for specifying security requirements of cryptographic modules that are a set of software, hardware or firmware to implement approved security functions, which include the algorithm and key generation. Healthcare and other regulated industries that collect, store, share, transfer and disseminate sensitive information, must use the cryptographic modules produced by private sector or open source communities.

FIPS 140-2 is the most current version of the standard as documented by NIST or the National Institute of Standards and Technology. FIPS establishes CMVP or the Cryptographic Module Validation Program, which is a joint effort by NIST and CSE or Communications Security Establishment of Canada.

The National Voluntary Laboratory Accreditation Program has accredited 13 third-party laboratories as cryptographic module testing laboratories for handling CMVP testing. Modules are tested here against the security requirements of FIPS 140-2 and cover 11 areas, including implementation of algorithms approved by FIPS, generation of random numbers through approved methods, specified management of the lifecycle of the decryption key and self-testing.

Within these areas, the cryptographic module under test receives a rating for security level from 1-4, depending on the requirements that it could meet. A module receives FIPS 140-2 validations only for a specific version of the software program running on a particular version of hardware.

CONCLUSION

While any vendor can claim to provide system security since it uses the best encryption technology available, you are likely to risk exposure with systems unable to meet the FIPS 140-2 standard for information encryption. Armed with the FIPS validation process, healthcare systems can manage the security of their critical data with a new level of confidence.

TEXT MESSAGING COMPLIANCE & HIPAA

Although sending unencrypted text messages involves significant risks of noncompliance with HIPAA and other acts, the method is a fast and convenient way to communicate.

There can be significant risks involved with transmitting Electronic Protected Health Information or ePHI using unencrypted text messaging, especially with the increasing pressure of enforcing the compliance with HITECH and HIPAA. On the other hand, healthcare providers see text messaging as a fast and convenient way to collaborate and communicate with colleagues.

THE COMPLIANCE MANDATE OF HIPAA AND HITECH

According to the HIPAA Security Rule, organizations must address text messaging as a part of their management strategy and carry out a comprehensive risk analysis. Depending on the outcome of the risk analysis, the organization must decide on the appropriate technical, physical and administrative controls that will mitigate the risks of using text messaging for sending ePHI.

Before the healthcare organization can decide on the necessary technical security measures that it requires for complying with this standard, it must review the current methods it is using for transmitting ePHI. As a next step, it has to identify the means available as well as appropriate for protecting ePHI and select a suitable solution. The healthcare organization can send adequately protected ePHI an over open, electronic network, without violating the Security Rule.

HITECH requires healthcare organizations to notify patients in cases of breach of ePHI. Texting impacts this area of compliance as well. The HIPAA Final Rule defines "breach" as the disclosure, use, access or acquisition of PHI in a manner not permitted by the HIPAA Privacy Rule, which compromises the privacy or security of such information.

Typically, texting involves use of devices such as tablets and smartphones and these can potentially be lost or stolen. Therefore, it is important that healthcare organizations review and ensure HITECH compliance in the event of a breach when the text message resides on such a compromised device.

POLICY SHOULD INCLUDE TEXT MESSAGING

Use of text messaging must be a part of the policy of the healthcare organization. Effectively, the scope should include all employees, physicians and affiliates. In addition, a Business Associate Agreement or BAA may be required for including third parties such as vendors and contractors to abide by parts of the policy of the organization. Moreover, the policy must cover all applications, systems and networks that process, store or transmit ePHI and other sensitive information.

For establishing the minimal requirements in the organization, its policy for secure text messaging should include key statements such as:

- Text messages are electronic communications. A computer or a mobile device may be used to transmit text messages, which may include written words, videos and photos. When the content of such a message contains ePHI, the text message must comply with HIPAA requirements.

- Only an approved, encrypted and secure format must be used for transmitting any text message containing ePHI.

REQUIREMENTS TO BE MET IN THE POLICY

When transmitting, storing or processing ePHI using a text messaging application, certain requirements must be met, such as:

Before sending any text message containing ePHI, users must make sure that the application will encrypt the message during both transit and while at rest. The mobile provider or a software program must encrypt the message when sending it from the sending device to the recipient's device. The cellular provider must not store the encrypted or decrypted text message on their systems in ways that it is accessible to an unauthorized person.

When employees wish to send ePHI via text messages to other employees, all senders and receivers must fulfill encryption requirements for messages both in transit and at rest.

Employees sending or receiving text messages containing ePHI, must make sure that they are using a secure text application approved by the IT department as suitable for the purpose. Employees must submit their mobile numbers for a proper inventory to be maintained by the IT department.

It is necessary to properly sanitize any retired mobile device that was used for texting ePHI. The IT department must wipe all mobile devices securely when they are returned. Employees using personal devices must contact the IT department and have their devices securely wiped prior to returning it to their cellular provider.

To be effective, the policy enforcing the use of secure text messaging must mandate safeguards to be implemented by employees who wish to send or receive messages. These safeguards must include:

- Password protection for the mobile device or the secure texting application; the user should never disable this feature.

- Automatic lock enabled after a period of inactivity not exceeding five minutes.

- Limiting to the minimum necessary information when texting messages with ePHI—multiple factors identifying the patient must not be used

To ensure accuracy of the information being texted, some precautions must be administered. The following guidelines must be followed when texting ePHI:

- Before sending, confirm presence of the recipient

- Recipient must confirm reception of the message

- Do not use abbreviations or shorthand

- Be careful about using auto-correction functions; review text for accuracy prior to sending

- Do not text patient orders

- Make sure that all text messages used for clinical decision making are documented in medical records

- If the information is no longer needed, delete all text messages containing ePHI as early as possible

Based on the compliance mandate of specific organizations, policy statements to be considered and adopted may include:

- All unencrypted text messages with ePHI received or sent out must be immediately reported to the IT department or to the HIPAA Security Officer

- Any text message sent to a wrong individual must be reported to the IT department or to the HIPAA Security Officer

- Maintain every revision of a policy and procedure for a minimum period of six years from the date of its creation or when it was last in effect, whichever is later

- Maintain all logs relevant to security incidents and log-in audit information for a period of six years

REQUIREMENTS TO BE MET BY A SECURE TEXTING SOLUTION

For ensuring compliance with HIPAA requirements, and enable employees to use text messaging securely, healthcare organizations must work with vendors that meet the following key capabilities:

Authentication methods: End-to-end secure authentication methods and environment methods must be provided to ensure authorized access

Password management: Generation and use of sufficiently complex passwords along with secure mechanisms for change/reset

Administrator rights: Must be separate from regular user rights

Login monitoring: Must log and monitor all attempts, both successful and failures. Must lock the account after a defined number of failed login attempts

Access control: Users must have access only to the messages they have sent or received Logging of all administrative access and actions including resetting of administrative passwords for users

Automatic logoff: Must log out the user from the application after a period of inactivity

Unique user identification: Users must be uniquely identified throughout the application and it must be possible to tie all actions directly to these IDs

Access control audits: Must be able to generate reports on access controls, including actions of administrators

Account authorization and establishment: Only administrators must have the ability to create new accounts. Must log all account creation and modifications

Account termination: Only an administrator should be able to terminate an account Terminated accounts must not be able to access any previous messages and must not be able to send any new message

Audit capabilities: Must log all user actions related to message actions and authentication, must log all administrative access related to elevated access activities and managing users, must time-stamp all logs for easier correlation

Transmission security: Must ensure that the data is protected while in transit. The transmission security provided must be independent of the transmitting platform

Data protection on the mobile device: Messages stored on mobile devices must be encrypted independent of any native device encryption. All proprietary data cached on the device must also be encrypted. Encryption algorithm must conform to industry standard AES256. Resetting the application password must destroy all saved messages

Backup processes: All messages must be archived for allowing administrative access. Archived messages must be encrypted and stored securely. Third party storage must not have access to archived ePHI. Message retention times must be customizable to meet the requirements of the organizational policy. Access to message archives must be restricted

Cloud-hosted solution: Solution must be a cloud-hosted SaaS that does not require on-premise hardware or infrastructure

Secure photo sharing: Must allow photos to be taken and attached to text messages. Sharing or accessing outside the texting application must not be possible

Texting across multiple organizations: A single application must allow texting across multiple organizations. Users with multiple accounts can have a contact directory and a unified inbox

Notifications and read receipts: Must provide notifications and read receipts as visual indication and time stamp

Callback requests: Must embed phone number directly into the message to enable callback with a single tap

Streamlined contact directory: Must allow users to search, find and text all contacts in the application directory, without typing any phone number. Administrators must be able to populate the contact directory

Customizable sounds: Must allow users to set the tone of the sound alert when a new message is received.

ADMINISTRATIVE REQUIREMENTS TO BE MET BY A SECURE TEXTING SOLUTION

Active Directory synchronization: Must be able to add/remove/modify users directly. Administrators must be able to setup the synchronization without referring to the vendor

Secure notification: Message notifications displayed must not contain any ePHI

Remote wipe: Administrator must be able to disable accounts, revoking access to all messages and information

Preventing ePHI leakage: Incorrect entry of PIN on the mobile device for a certain number of times must destroy all saved data

Maintain organizational privacy: must not allow third parties to access ePHI

Set message life span: Administrator must be able to set how long messages will persist within an application on the device

Optional application PIN: Administrator must be able to set additional PIN on the application.

THE PRACTICE OF TRACKING AND MONITORING

With the deployment of a secure text messaging solution, ensuring active management is critical for maintaining compliance with HITECH and HIPAA requirements. This includes regular monitoring of log files and audit information for ensuring appropriate use. IT administrators must regularly:

- Track and monitor activities related to managing policies and users

- Ensure that all authentication events are captured appropriately

- Ensure that message read receipts have a time stamp

In addition, healthcare organizations must ensure that their proactive audit practice is aligned with the established policy and is implemented for managing the secure and HIPAA-compliant text-messaging framework.

BEST PRACTICES FOR VDT ACCESS AND PRIVACY

The law permits sharing of medical information related to the patient with his/her friends, family and legal personal representative, provided the information is relevant to treatment.

For patients who are able to permit explicitly the sharing of their PHI with "others", the current view, download and transmit or VDT regulatory requirements need best practice recommendations rather than an additional policy. The "others" being family, friends and personal representatives—designations defined by state law. Legal personal representatives may directly access the PHI of the patient if they have the legal rights, since under HIPAA, legal personal representatives can stand in for their patient with respect to accessing PHI.

The above is the view of the Privacy and Security Tiger Team, which presented its final recommendations on the VDT access to the HIT Policy Committee on April 8, 2014. The committee approved the recommendations of the Tiger Team.

Although not a requirement, the Privacy Rule allows covered entities to share their patients' PHI with members of the patients' family or other persons involved in the healthcare or payment for care of the individual. While individuals do have the right to object to such disclosures, they can also accomplish VDT access on their own simply by sharing their usernames and passwords.

It is not possible to control whether patients will decide to share their user names and passwords for granting VDT access, this is not advisable. It is very important to educate patients about why this is not advisable because, when patients grant VDT access on their own there is no way for the healthcare organization to keep track of who has taken action in VDT.

In order to combat these tendencies, the Tiger Team suggests that the process of granting credentials to authorized family, friends and personal representatives must be made sufficiently easy for discouraging shared access. At the same time, it must also sufficiently satisfy the need of assuring authorization and authentication/identification. The Tiger Team has advised the ONC or Office of the National Coordinator to accomplish developing and disseminating best practices for assuring that friends, family and where appropriate, legal personal representatives of adult patients, be allowed access to VDT.

The Tiger Team has forwarded five VDT best practices for ONC to consider. The first best practice, Authorization of Family/Friends, has been divided into two segments—easy and hard hypotheticals.

The easiest case is when a patient makes a request for VDT access for a family member or a friend:

- The patient makes the request in person or from remote. For example, over the phone, through VDT or via e-mail

- Healthcare providers must document that request. It would be helpful if the request can be stored electronically

- Providers can use out-of-band notification for notification/confirmation

The above is important, since a patient request for proxy access may also come remotely or through a software that is acting on behalf of the patient.

The more difficult case is when a family member or a friend makes the request or if the patient is incapacitated:

- It is necessary to confirm such request with the patient, possibly through out-of-band confirmation

- According to HIPAA, sharing of treatment-related information with family and friends is allowed, provided it is limited to only information relevant to treatment

- The healthcare provider is required to consider whether providing access to relevant information via VDT us the most appropriate vehicle

The next best practice suggested was the authorization of personal representatives. Since it depends on state law whether someone qualifies as a personal representative, and since the state law varies so much, it is very hard to form uniform recommendations for national policy or best practices. According to the Tiger Team, healthcare providers must review their methods of adapting their current VDT processes for granting personal representatives access to records. As a helpful capability, the healthcare organizations should also develop the ability of storing documentation related to status of the personal representative, including the patients' authorization of access by family/friends.

The best practices suggested for identity proofing and authentication were:

- The patient can either provide credentials or authorize the access directly (for example, via VDT or by communicating the contact information separately)

- Best practices suggested earlier for identity proofing and authentication

- The need to develop the capability and processes for cutting off VDT access by family, friends and personal representatives because of a change in preference by the patient or changes in the legal status of the personal representative

The best practices offered with respect to the scope of VDT access were:

- As VDT accounts can be programmed to offer more than "all or nothing" access for proxies with respect to both data content and function performed, it is very important to educate patients on the options available. This allows the patient to make informed decisions about the scope of the access to be granted to family/friends. When the option is limited to all or nothing, patients must be educated on the scope of information that anyone can access, if provided with proxy access.

- There is a need to determine whether VDT access to the personal representative will be limited to what can be legally accessible by the personal representative. Failing this, VDT access to personal representative must not be granted.

The best practices offered on continuing education of patients and providers were:

- ONC must disseminate best practices among healthcare providers. This will enable them to establish and/or remove proxy access to VDT accounts, maintaining consistency with needs of the patient and the law.

- Healthcare providers must also educate their patients on the benefits and risks involved with VDT. This education must be consistent with the prior recommendations of the HIT-PC, and must include the risks/benefits of proxy access.

STRATEGIES FOR PROTECTING PATIENT PRIVACY

On average, annually, two million Americans fall victim to medical identity theft and this costs the US healthcare organizations an estimated $41 billion.

Healthcare institutes are finding that it is getting increasingly difficult to comply with patient privacy regulations. As it is, the journey to a complete electronic health record is in itself a daunting task, and the constant changes to the patient privacy regulations are not making it any easier. After the enactment of the HIPAA Privacy statute in 1996, there have been several regulations regarding patient privacy—HITECH, ARRA Meaningful Use and the Omnibus Rule.

Patient privacy breaches in hospitals attract severe penalties, including criminal, financial and harm to reputation. The recent Omnibus Rule, with its tighter regulations, has complicated matters further. The audits from OCR have increased, and the press regularly carries headlines that most organizations entrusted with PHI protection are seldom upholding their responsibility.

When the stakes are so high, hospitals need to move beyond the random manual audits that they currently have in place. Especially since these audits review only a very small percentage of the access events taking place daily in the healthcare setting. A solid foundation is necessary—involving policy, procedures, and technology—for ensuring patient privacy throughout the healthcare organization.

TOP CHALLENGES IN SECURING PATIENT PRIVACY DATA

Although Healthcare is the most regulated industry in the US today, it is also the largest target for theft and fraud related to personal information and this threat is continuing to grow. An estimated 2 million Americans are victims of theft related to medical identity, which costs the healthcare organizations nearly $41 billion each year.

As lawmakers and healthcare consumers wrestle with this, as a result more regulations are likely and they will place an increased burden on IT organizations.

The Omnibus Rule and Meaningful Use have privacy requirements that HIPAA already touches upon:

- According to the Omnibus Rule, organizations are presumed guilty of a breach until they have proved their innocence with a four-step risk assessment.

- According to the Meaningful Use, organizations must conduct a risk analysis conforming to HIPAA 45 CFR 164.308(a)(1). This is identified as the Security Management Process.

As the cost of breaches and non-compliances rise sharply, privacy is now a business imperative. This is enhanced by the new regulations of the Omnibus Rule around breach notification, which make it very clear that hospitals must provide timely and accurate monitoring of access to patient records.

In complying with the strict regulations in order to avoid stiff penalties, healthcare organizations face three primary challenges in protecting patient data:

1. Logging every access to patient data

2. Auditing massive volumes of access records

3. Correlating diverse data into one database

To conform to HIPAA, healthcare providers have to log every access to patient data. However, use of electronic health records, improvements in data integration and increased networking now churn out massive amounts of data, which is again shared across several local and remote locations. Not only does this increase the number of data access points tremendously, it creates new challenges for protecting patient privacy. Currently, patient privacy requirements already span the many existing systems. In the future, this will increase as new systems such as physician portals and HIEs continue to be developed. Unless IT has developed a solid patient privacy foundation, they may not be able to bring these new systems online.

The volume of data that hospitals need to audit is enormous and a challenge in and of itself. For example, a hospital with a 100-bed facility, wanting to identify inappropriate access to the data of patients at their facility, has to audit 52,000 patient access records every day. Clearly, the task to find those that are inappropriate, by monitoring and reviewing these access records manually every day is simply not feasible.

Correlating the data from all logs across all different systems into one consolidated database is the third challenge. For this, the hospital must be able to see all the accesses across all systems in one go and thereby make it possible to detect trends and patterns including the magnitude of the privacy violations.

CONSEQUENCES OF CURRENT PRACTICES

A report commissioned by the Kroll Advisory Solutions reveals that not many hospitals are focused on patient privacy and that health-care organizations do not allocate appropriate resources or focus specifically to ensure that all patient health information remains secure and protected. The report found that:

- 47% of the healthcare organizations spend less than 3% of their IT budgets on security of information
- 66% audit regularly for internal breach and disclosure
- 11% reported a case of medical identity theft
- 91% review their audit logs and 84% of them review it manually

That leads to many questions being asked, such as:

- Why are healthcare organizations not fully implementing preventive measures for a data breach?
- Why are healthcare organizations performing only random audits?
- Why are healthcare organizations not taking advantage of creating better policies and processes and or seeking technological advantages to reduce the cost of manual effort?

It seems that the fundamental problem lies in the lack of understanding regarding privacy violations and the potential consequences. Once healthcare leaders truly understand the extent of inappropriate PHI access in their facilities, understand the privacy expectations of their patients and understand the ramifications, they would reallocate their resources.

In addition, most healthcare organizations do not have appropriate staff in place to maintain the privacy program. Usually, patient privacy is a secondary or tertiary job for employees, who are unclear about responsibilities and requirements that their state and government expects of them.

Such a lack of preparedness can lead to serious consequences. The new Omnibus Rule and the HITECH mandate require hospitals to notify patients within 60 days if their PHI has been inappropriately accessed. Some states require even tighter reporting. Organizations that fail to comply can face penalties up to $1.5 million in a year. The same rule applies whether it is a case of identity theft, active snooping, theft for profit or a careless mistake. Ignorance of the breach or of the law can no longer be forwarded as a defense. In fact, authorities may identify it as "willful neglect", which carries with it stiff civil and sometimes, criminal penalties.

A THREE-STEP METHODOLOGY CAN LEAD TO A SOLID FOUNDATION

A patient privacy compliance program with three elements can provide a solid foundation that can also reduce the risk of a data breach:

- Policies
- Procedures
- Technology

POLICIES

When healthcare organizations accept and understand the importance of patient privacy, it will then be reflected in their policies. Typically, a committee forms the privacy policies of the organization. The committee may include the Human Resources, CFO, CIO, security officer, patient privacy officer and the compliance officer. The HITRUST Common Security Framework has some models that healthcare organizations can use to help create their policy.

PROCEDURES

To enforce the policy, healthcare organizations need to move to the next phase. This involves development of processes for developing, documenting, implementing and communicating procedures that will enforce the conditions set forth in their privacy policy. In not setting up diligent procedures for monitoring what employees are doing, healthcare organizations will inadvertently set themselves up for failure and embarrassment.

Most surprisingly, the real threat comes from within. The current healthcare practice model actually encourages open access to all caregivers, who can access all patient information. When applied to people working in the emergency department, this makes sense, as limiting their access to patient records can only hamper patient care.

Therefore, essentially, healthcare personnel do have access to everything that is appropriate, but they are not allowed to look at everything. This can complicate the enforcement of patient privacy procedures—caregivers need access to all the information, but then someone has to check the audit logs to make sure they indeed accessed only the required information.

TECHNOLOGY

Technology is necessary to perform certain tasks which cannot be addressed quite as efficiently if done manually. Hospitals and healthcare organizations can now move beyond the limitations of random and manual audits, since with the appropriate technology, they can automate monitoring of patient privacy.

For example, with the Iatric Systems Security Audit Manager, the healthcare organization can perform proactive 100% privacy protection to make a real-time review of all user interaction with patient information. So in a hospital setting, this can mean a comprehensive and immediate breach detection and notification.

Implementing automation via technology helps healthcare organizations in investigating and tracking a breach more easily. They can generate reports on any unauthorized access to the medical records of a patient and put practices in place to prevent the breach from happening again. Any automated solution for integrating and correlating access to PHI located in multiple healthcare systems is the simplest and most effective way to streamline all processes and procedures for ensuring compliance. The OCR HIPAA audits and the Omnibus Rule make it necessary for the healthcare organizations to have practices in place that can not only prove that the hospital is capable of monitoring access to patient records, but also it is able to do something about a breach when detected.

A TECHNOLOGY CHECKLIST FOR PROTECTING PHI

When evaluating technology for a patient privacy-monitoring program, a checklist makes sure that the selected system is capable of offering the critical capabilities:

- **Central monitoring of all accesses to patient records:** By automatically aggregating audit logs from across the entire organization and providing single search queries and proactive auditing

- **Catching and resolving single as well as recurring breaches in real-time:** It is important that inappropriate activity be spotted as it happens by proactively auditing all access to patient records

- **Documenting breach investigations and their resolution:** With a centralized and automated system, information required for documenting all investigation and their resolutions can be easily provided for fulfilling notification requirements

- **Providing reporting per state and federal guidelines:** Helps in the creation of a centralized, comprehensive environment for reviewing documented findings and providing insight into areas that require additional security measures and/or employee education

- **Documenting the release of medical records**b When releasing medical records, a HIPAA violation can occur in so many ways and it is important that there is a procedure in place to document and track their release

- **Accounting for all disclosures:** Hospitals and business associates are required to account for all disclosures of PHI, and the process must be able to track and document the disclosures in a central repository

- **Meeting Meaningful Use requirements of patient privacy:** Should allow hospitals to implement policies and procedures for preventing, detecting, containing and correcting security violations under HIPAA 45 CFR 164.308(a)(1).

THE COST AND COMPLEXITY INVOLVED WITH ENDPOINT MANAGEMENT

Limited budget should not be a constraint for mid-sized organizations to improve on endpoint security, patch compliance, and lifecycle management.

Although headlines usually highlight security attacks on larger entities, cyber criminals are shifting their focus to midsized organizations as well. The reasons are not hard to find, with limited budgets and IT staff, but a growing amount of valuable information, these SMBs present a highly attractive target.

The true cost of these security breaches is not limited to just revenue loss, inadequate compliance or compromised data. Incidents of security could result in a loss of trust among consumers, suppliers and partners. The organization's reputation may also be damaged for years to come and may even result in its failure.

Simultaneously, preventing breaches of security is becoming increasingly challenging. Organizations have to depend on a large number of physical and virtual endpoints, which include servers, self-service kiosks, ATMs, POS devices, smartphones and tablets, laptops and desktops. While running different operating systems and applications, these disparate devices often access the network from remote locations. All this leads to compliance gaps, missing patches and configuration errors. With traditional safeguards, it is impossible to keep up with the latest threats.

On the other hand, SMBs have to combat the increasing sophistication of malicious crooks when their IT budgets are constantly shrinking. Fortunately, a single, cost-effective solution for endpoint management is available to help SMBs improve their security, visibility and patch compliance, and all within a limited IT budget.

ENDPOINT MANAGEMENT CAN THWART ATTACKS

Traditionally, SMBs have depended upon manual processes for patching, managing and securing their diverse endpoints. However, as the organization grows and uses increasingly distributed environments, the manual processes can be hard to sustain. This leads to the endpoints becoming the weakest links in the IT security chain, inviting more attacks. New types of spyware and worms, including malicious viruses, are directed towards the organization, and security admins often have to deal with potential threats hidden within web pages and emails.

Working remotely or from branch offices with practically no IT staff onsite, is another challenge as organizations expand. Such employees may not have access to secure internet connections, and may not be connecting with a VPN. All this makes it critical for the organization to invest in effective endpoint management and protect itself, regardless of how the endpoint is connected or where it is located.

BUSINESS RESULTS EXPECTED FROM ENDPOINT MANAGEMENT

Real-world studies with deployments of endpoint management have turned up encouraging results:

- Reduction in labor costs—50%

- Increase in compliance rate for patches and updates—98%

- Reduction in calls to the helpdesk—50%

- Reduction in patch compliance times—80%

- Increase in first-pass success rate of patching—50 to 99%

- Malware infections after implementation—None

HOW IS PATCH MANAGEMENT SIMPLIFIED?

Endpoints, whether they are used in the office or at a remote location, can be the attack points leading to exposure if they have configuration errors and or lack critical patches. SMBs may not be able to deploy security patches rapidly in such cases. Some resort to free patch management products, but that may be expensive overall, requiring more infrastructure and IT staff to manage them. Moreover, the free tools are usually OS-centric and unable to protect common third-party applications.

With single-source patch management solutions, SMBs need only mid-sized budgets to manage a constant flow of patches. IT admins can apply the proper patch to the correct endpoint and even verify that the patch is effectively applied. Such solutions support continuous patch compliance with automatic enforcement of patch policies.

The simplified patch management solution offers many advantages to SMBs:

- Automatic patch management for multiple OS and applications covering a wide range of endpoints, irrespective of their status, connection types and location

- Greater visibility into patch compliance leading to flexible and near real-time reporting and monitoring

- Single console visibility of patch status for all endpoints

- Reduction in security risk as streamlining the remediation cycles takes hours and not weeks

- Patching online and offline virtual machines improves security in virtual environments

- Patching endpoints either on or off the network, including those using Internet connections and other roaming devices, implying they receive patches with minimal impact

- Improvement in audit readiness because of simple and fast compliance reports

IMPROVEMENTS IN LIFECYCLE MANAGEMENT

As businesses expand, the number and types of endpoints also explode and it becomes more essential to have tools for managing their lifecycles. With cost-effective and easy-to-deploy key lifecycle management capabilities, SMBs can handle software distribution and automate the process of asset discovery.

Not limited to automating patch management, these solutions provide visibility of all connections to the network, including the software installed. Within a single console, administrators can discover and inventory the resources, distribute and manage applications for different systems and OS. They can empower end users to deploy necessary applications using self-service portals.

Available lifecycle management solutions let SMBs attain high levels of automation together with fine-grained configuration management, allowing them to:

- Scan their entire network in a distributed manner for identifying all IP-addressable devices, including routers and switches, printers, other peripherals, network devices and computing endpoints

- Automate the software distribution across workstations and servers with different OS, using a software package library featuring high performance

- Allow end-users a self-service portal for deploying approved and available software

- Enforce and manage password policies for protecting the security of local user accounts

- Use group membership to create operator accounts

- Use automated system updates and patching to address the entire endpoint lifecycle

- Reduce the expense and clutter of tools that multiple vendors introduce

ENSURING COMPLIANCE

Cyber criminals are not the only concern of SMBs with security gaps. Stakeholders, general public, suppliers and regulatory agencies all demand compliance with the latest privacy and security requirements.

Government regulations also require many SMBs to establish, document and prove compliance with security policies. For operating as a supplier to larger enterprises, SMBs now require to demonstrate proof of compliance as a part of the contracting process.

Endpoint management solutions help SMBs to enforce security policies while reporting on compliance quickly, thus improving their audit preparedness. Such solutions help the IT staff to:

- Locate and fix real-time issues related to the health, compliance status and currency of popular anti-virus products from different third parties for a variety of operating systems

- Ensure automation of configuration for endpoint security management

- Automate customized quarantine rules for isolating out-of-compliance endpoints or malware attacks until remediation is found

- Identify advanced persistent threats and respond within minutes, regardless of the location or type of endpoint

- Simplify the deployment of various security products

- Discover all IP-enabled assets and report on them, even when they are across heterogeneous OS

CONCLUSION

Affordable solutions are available for SMBs to improve their endpoint security, lifecycle management and patch compliance. Single, key solutions such as the Endpoint Manager family from reputed organizations such as IBM help to reduce the cost and burden on IT staff, while providing continuous visibility, control, and compliance of endpoints.

Made in the USA
Middletown, DE
02 March 2018